Pharmacy OSCEs

T0187027

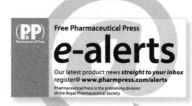

Pharmacy OSCEs

A revision guide

Edited by

Beti Wyn Evans
BPharm, DipClinPharm, PGC (Higher Education), MRPharmS

Laura Kravitz
BSc, Cert Psych Th, PGC (Higher Education), FHEA, MRPharmS

Kelly Lefteri
BPharm (Hons), PGClinDip, MEd, FHEA, MRPharmS

Nina Walker
MPharm, PGC (Higher Education), PgDip, FHEA, MRPharmS

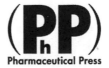

Pharmaceutical Press

Published by the Pharmaceutical Press

66-68 East Smithfield, London E1W 1AW, UK

© Royal Pharmaceutical Society of Great Britain 2012

(PP) is a trade mark of Pharmaceutical Press

Pharmaceutical Press is the publishing division of the Royal
Pharmaceutical Society

First published 2013
Reprinted 2014, 2016, 2017, 2020, 2021, 2023

Typeset by Laserwords Private Limited, Chennai, India
Printed in Great Britain by TJ Books Limited, Padstow, Cornwall

ISBN 978 0 85711 0435

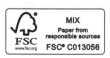

Contents

Acknowledgement

The editors acknowledge staff and students of the University of Hertfordshire.

About the editors

Beti Wyn Evans BPharm, DipClinPharm, PGC (Higher Education), MRPharmS, is principal lecturer in pharmacotherapeutics at the University of Hertfordshire. Beti has a background in hospital pharmacy with experience in clinical pharmacy and medicines information. In academia, Beti has experience of undergraduate and postgraduate education of pharmacists, prescribing advice and systematic reviewing, including developing NICE clinical guidelines.

Laura Kravitz BSc, Cert Psych Th, PGC (Higher Education), FHEA, MRPharmS, is principal lecturer in clinical pharmacy and Programme Tutor at the University of Hertfordshire, Department of Pharmacy. Her research interests include OSCE and she has published in this area. Prior to joining the staff at the university, Laura was a mental health pharmacist, with particular interest in the treatment of early episode schizophrenia.

Kelly Lefteri BPharm (Hons), PGClinDip, MEd, FHEA, MRPharmS, is a principal lecturer and Deputy Head of Pharmacy Practice at the University of Hertfordshire. She has a background in community pharmacy, education and management and is involved in teaching undergraduate and postgraduate students the fundamentals of pharmacy practice. Prior to joining the university, Kelly was a pre-registration learning and development manager.

Nina Walker MPharm, PGC (Higher Education), PgDip, FHEA, MRPharmS, is a principal lecturer in pharmacy practice at the University of Hertfordshire. She is a qualified pharmacist who completed her MPharm degree at the University of

Nottingham and then went on to completed her Diploma in Pharmacy Practice at the School of Pharmacy, London. Her interests include simulated learning, numeracy development and student engagement. Nina's background is hospital pharmacy focusing on medicines management and education and training.

About the authors

Narinder Bhalla BSc (Hons) Pharmacy, MSc in Pharmacy Practice, Independent Prescriber (IP), splits his time between the University of Hertfordshire Department of Pharmacy and Cambridge University of Hertfordshire NHS Foundation Trust. Within the hospital trust Narinder holds the post of Consultant Pharmacist – Medication Safety with a key role in strategically managing and implementing medication safety solutions across the trust. His clinical specialty area is cardiovascular medicine. At the university, Narinder holds the post of teacher practitioner and has contributed to the development of postgraduate masters programmes for pharmacists as well as a number of modules related to a range of clinical areas.

Matthew Catterall Pg Cert, BSc (Hons), Dip HCP (ECP), Dip IMC (RCSEd), FHEA, MCPara is a senior lecturer and post-qualification undergraduate programme lead in paramedic science at the University of Hertfordshire. Matthew has a clinical background as a paramedic, previously practising as a paramedic practitioner and advanced paramedic. He has teaching experience on pre- and post-registration degree programmes for paramedics and is the curriculum development lead for paramedics' professional organisation, the College of Paramedics. Currently he is completing the dissertation component of a MSc in Cardiology and Education, investigating clinical reasoning used by paramedics while managing heart failure.

John Donaghy BSc (Hons), Pg Cert, Fellow HEA, FCPara is principal lecturer and professional lead for paramedic science, School of Health and Social Work, University of Hertfordshire, and is responsible for the development and delivery of the paramedic programmes at the university. John's current academic and training role follows over 30 years' service with the London Ambulance Service, before moving into higher education. John is a Council member of the Health Professions Council (HPC) and is currently undertaking a Professional Doctorate in Education. His research interests lie predominantly in qualitative analysis and his current work explores student acculturation into the ambulance service.

Cathal Gallagher BPharm, MA, LLM, PhD, is principal lecturer in pharmacy practice at the University of Hertfordshire.

Sarah Jardine BSc (Hons), PGCE, FHEA, is principal lecturer and programme lead for paramedic science at the University of Hertfordshire. Sarah has a clinical background as both a physiotherapist and a paramedic and teaches mainly in the areas of patient assessment, minor injury and chronic illness.

Andrzej Kostrzewski MSc, MMedEd, PhD, MRPharmS, FHEA, is the academic lead for clinical development, University of Hertfordshire, Hatfield, UK. He is also the academic lead for clinical pharmacy at the Department of Pharmacy, University of Hertfordshire. He has extensive experience of education and training, and is an experienced clinical practitioner with over 25 years' experience in hospital practice and holds a current clinical attachment with Guy's & St Thomas' NHS Foundation Trust.

Paul Power MA (UCL), BSc (Hons), Adv Dip Health Service Research, AGSM, RN, is senior lecturer in paramedic science, teaching on undergraduate and postgraduate paramedic science and interprofessional programmes. With a clinical background in anaesthetics and resuscitation he has held senior clinical and educational positions in a number of major London teaching hospitals and Addenbrooke's Hospital Cambridge before working full time in higher education. He is currently reading for a Doctorate in Education, with a special interest in developing clinical reasoning for paramedics.

John R Purvis BPharm, PhD, Cert Vet Pharm, FHEA, is professor of pharmacy education at the University of Bradford. John holds a PhD in pharmacology, and has experience of community pharmacy practice. His extensive academic roles have included the first lectureship in clinical pharmacy in the UK that incorporated both academic and community pharmacy components; Professor of Pharmacy Education; Associate Dean (Learning and Teaching) for the School of Life Sciences at the University of Bradford and, from 2004 to 2008, Head of the Bradford School of Pharmacy. John has many years' experience as an external examiner at a number of UK schools of pharmacy, and is a member of the Modernising Pharmacy Careers Programme Board. John's particular interests in pharmacy education include: curriculum design; learner-centred approaches to education; strategies for enhancing the learning and assessment of clinical reasoning, clinical decision-making and consultation skills. John has been designing and using OSCEs in undergraduate pharmacy education since 1988.

Aamer Safdar BPharm (Hons), MSc, PGCE, MA, FHEA, is principal pharmacist lead for education and development at Guy's and St Thomas', London, where he has a wide range of educational and managerial responsibilities. His main interest is in pre-registration training and is involved with teaching and tutoring students at postgraduate and undergraduate levels and is involved with courses at Diploma and Masters levels, including the MSc in Clinical Pharmacy International Practice and Policy with the UCL School of Pharmacy. Aamer lectures at King's College London and has completed a National Leadership Academy Clinical Leadership Fellowship which incorporates a PG Certificate in Leadership and Service Improvement.

Jennifer Silverthorne is clinical senior lecturer in the School of Pharmacy and Pharmaceutical Sciences at the University of Manchester. She is programme director for the Postgraduate Diploma in Clinical and Health Services Pharmacy and leads the clinical teaching of pharmacy undergraduates. Jennifer is also a part-time hospital pharmacist providing a clinical service to Elderly Care wards at Salford Royal NHS Trust. She obtained her BPharm degree from the University of Bath before undertaking a postgraduate clinical diploma at the University of Manchester and an MEd in Clinical Education at the University of Leeds.

John Talbot BSc (Hons) is senior lecturer in paramedic science and emergency care practitioner. John has a background in out of hospital care as a paramedic and emergency care practitioner as well as lecturing in biosciences, patient assessment and management and pharmacology at the University of Hertfordshire.

Gary Venstone BSc (Hons), PGCE, FHEA, is a senior lecturer in paramedic science at the University of Hertfordshire. Gary has a clinical background as a paramedic and emergency care practitioner and has many years' experience in Ambulance Service training and education. With a particular interest in patient examination and assessment Gary teaches on both pre- and post-registration degree programmes for paramedics.

Julia Williams PhD, PGCE, HFCPara, FHEA, is a principal lecturer and research lead for paramedic science at the University of Hertfordshire, and an Adjunct Associate Professor at the Queensland University of Technology in the School of Clinical Sciences. Julia has a clinical background in critical care and has extensive experience of undertaking healthcare research as well as teaching research methods and practice on pre- and post-registration degree programmes for paramedics.

Abbreviations

ACS	acute coronary syndrome
AED	automated external defibrillator
ALT	alanine transaminase
AST	aspartate transaminase
BMI	body mass index
BNF	*British National Formulary*
CD	controlled drug
CKS	Clinical Knowledge Summaries
COCP	combined oral contraceptive pill
COPD	chronic obstructive pulmonary disease
CPD	continuous professional development
DH	drug history
FH	family history
GCA	giant cell arteritis
GGT	gamma glutamyltransferase
GP	general practitioner
HDL	high-density lipoprotein
HPC	history of presenting complaint
ICU	intensive care unit
INR	international normalised ratio
IM	intramuscular
IV	intravenous
LDL	low-density lipoprotein
MDI	metered dose inhaler
MEP	*Medicines, Ethics and Practice*

MMR	measles, mumps, rubella
MOH	medication overuse headache
MRSA	methicillin-resistant *Staphylococcus aureus*
NaCl	sodium chloride
NHS	National Health Service
NICE	National Institute for Health and Clinical Excellence
NSAID	non-steroidal anti-inflammatory drug
OTC	over the counter
PC	presenting complaint
PCI	percutaneous coronary intervention
PIL	Patient Information Leaflet
PMH	past medical history
PMR	patient medication record
POM	prescription-only medicine
POP	progestogen-only pill
q.d.s.	four times daily
ROS	review of systems
SAH	subarachnoid haemorrhage
SH	social history
SOL	space-occupying lesion
SPC	Summary of Product Characteristics
SSRI	selective serotonin reuptake inhibitor
TB	tuberculosis
TG	triglyceride
TTH	tension-type headache
URTI	upper respiratory tract infection
UTI	urinary tract infection

Introduction

Laura Kravitz and John Purvis

The Objective Structured Clinical Examination (OSCE) has been a feature of medical school programmes since the 1970s. OSCEs were introduced to assess professional performance in practice within a safe environment, where neither student nor patient is at risk of harm. Clinical scenarios are simulated, the student responding as if they were a qualified health professional.

Some students find OSCEs a stressful form of assessment. The student is exposed to the direct scrutiny of members of staff and simulated patients or healthcare professionals. They have to find solutions to problems within a tight time-frame. Students who are well prepared for OSCEs tend to be calmer and this correlates with a stronger performance. Engagement with formative OSCEs will support students in their preparation for and performance in summative OSCEs.

The aim of this book is to prepare you for OSCEs, to give you the best opportunity to perform as well as possible. The authors of the book are all OSCE examiners and have extensive experience of writing OSCE scenarios.

Preparing for OSCE

What are OSCE stations likely to involve?

You can probably guess the topics which will be assessed by OSCE, they are likely to be the most challenging to test in other types of assessment. For example:

- responding to symptoms
- history-taking
- counselling patients about prescription medicines

- communicating information relating to medicines to healthcare professionals, patients or carers
- record-keeping
- problem-solving (e.g. identifying drug interactions or interpreting laboratory data and recommending appropriate management)
- dosage calculations
- advising about drug administration.

Ask yourself if you are *really* confident with the following topics. If not, spend time revising these areas:

- being able to interpret laboratory biochemical data
- monitoring requirements and understanding of results such as the international normalised ratio (INR)
- simple dosage calculations, such as dosages for children expressed as mg per kg or mg per m^2
- basic pharmacokinetics, more complex formulae will be supplied, but clearance or volume of distribution might be considered common knowledge.

Familiarise yourself with the reference sources

Chapter 4 of this book, 'Data retrieval and interpretation', covers the use of reference sources. Many of these reference sources are available online, perhaps through your university extranet service. While it is a good idea to practise using the online material, you must remember that you are going to be using the book version in the OSCE. The best time to start working out *Martindale*'s complex indexing system is certainly not during a 5-minute OSCE! Take some time to explore these books in the library. At a minimum, look at *Martindale*, *Stockley's Drug Interactions*, the *BNF* (*British National Formulary*) and the *BNF for Children*. Identify where particular information is located, so that you can retrieve material quickly. Similarly, have a look through some Patient Information Leaflets and Summary of Product Characteristics (available at www.medicines.org.uk/emc/, accessed 6 June 2012). These materials follow a specific format and you will save time if you know exactly where to look first.

The *BNF* deserves further mention. Most students need little encouragement to look at their *BNF* during OSCEs. Spend a little time becoming familiar with the edition of the *BNF* that you intend to take into the examination.

- Do you understand all the symbols? Remind yourself by flicking through the abbreviations page prior to the OSCEs (e.g. Advisory Committee on Borderline Substances (ACBS)).
- Remember that when looking at an individual citation for a drug, further information may be included in the class citation. For example, if you are looking for information about ibuprofen, there is more information at the beginning of 10.1.1 than in the individual monograph.
- Familiarise yourself with the location of the various 'equivalent dosages'. For example, look up equivalent benzodiazepines doses, this is located at the beginning of 4.1.1 Hypnotics. Similarly equivalent corticosteroid doses are found at the beginning of 6.3.2. However, finding equivalent dosages of morphine and diamorphine is less straightforward. This is not at the beginning of 4.7.2 Opioid analgesics, but within Prescribing in palliative care.
- Have a good look at the appendices in the *BNF* edition that you will be using. These are an accessible source of information. Older editions have separate appendices for hepatic failure, renal failure, pregnancy and breastfeeding. Newer copies have this information within the main body of the book.
- The *BNF* highlights very important information, such as warnings, by using a coloured box or different font. This is intended to draw the reader's eye. Some students ignore these during OSCEs!
- Many drugs are used for a number of clinical indications. The treatment schedule may vary considerably. For example, look at the dose of cyproterone used to treat acne, male hypersexuality and malignant disease.

Be careful to choose the most appropriate indication when using the index.

'Bell ringers'

As you develop your clinical skills you will be identifying some drugs which are tricky to use. For example they have narrow therapeutic indices, are enzyme inhibitors or inducers, need therapeutic drug monitoring or have very serious adverse effects. These are the medicines most likely to appear in OSCEs, they are also the ones most likely to cause problems in practice. These drugs could be called 'bell ringers', which is to say that when you encounter them bells start ringing in your head! You can probably think of a few immediately – digoxin, warfarin, methotrexate, carbamazepine and erythromycin.

Why not create revision aids for these drugs, in a suitable format? An example is provided in Figure 1.

Practise your communication, consultation and counselling skills

If you are not familiar with speaking to patients and other healthcare professionals about medication-related issues, it is possible to practise these skills at home. Try explaining the solutions to the scenarios in this book to friends or family.

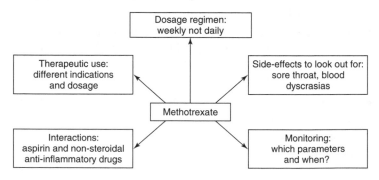

Figure 1   Revision aid for methotrexate.

This is particularly useful for helping you to understand the type of language that you should use with patients. You could print out a Patient Information Leaflet and try to explain how to use a device (such as an inhaler) to someone who has never used one, using a household prop! Your friends and family will certainly tell you if they don't understand. This method also works for complex dosage schemes, such as decreasing doses of steroid. Remember that in the OSCE the 'patient' may be a tutor, an actor or a member of the public from a voluntary organisation.

Consultation/communication skills are discussed in detail at the end of this introduction.

On the day of the OSCE

- Arrive in plenty of time. This sounds obvious, but OSCEs are stressful enough without adding to your worries. In many centres OSCEs run as an automated circuit and latecomers cannot be admitted.
- Remember to bring all necessary items. Your centre will tell you what you may bring, such as a calculator and a *BNF*.
- Dress appropriately. You may be advised of a dress code. Many students feel more confident when dressed as a professional would dress.

Approaching a new scenario

- Read the instructions carefully. Try to avoid jumping to conclusions. This is particularly important with the 'bell ringers' (see above). It is easy, especially if you are nervous, not to consider all the possible options. Once you have a plan, decide if you need to look up any information. Students sometimes waste valuable time looking up information that they actually know. Once you have decided what you need to look up, decide which of the available reference sources is the most appropriate.
- Remember that each scenario is a new start. Many students will dwell on previous scenarios that they found

difficult, to the detriment of their performance at further stations.

- OSCEs differ from other types of assessment in their ability to test a student's competence to communicate verbally. This means that there will be marks assigned to verbal communication. If appropriate, introduce yourself. Finish each station by asking if the patient/healthcare professional understands or if they have further questions. If you are given a patient name, use it.
- Try to maintain eye contact with the 'patient' or examiner. There may be marks assigned for non-verbal communication.
- Don't hide behind your *BNF* – it is a reference source not a defence system!
- Remember your mnemonics and apply them in their entirety. This is particularly important if you are nervous, it will stop you missing out vital questions.
- If the scenario begins with the patient/healthcare professional speaking, listen carefully to what they have to say. Try not to start rummaging in your *BNF* before they have finished speaking. If you are distracted you may miss vital information, it is also poor non-verbal communication.

How to use this book

Chapters of this book focus on different themes of OSCE scenarios. For example, if you are an undergraduate preparing for your dispensing assessments, you should find Chapter 3 very relevant; or if you are a postgraduate pharmacist studying for a prescribing qualification you may find Chapter 2 particularly useful. Scenarios are of varying complexity, ranging from early undergraduate years through to postgraduate. The suggested years of study for which the station may be appropriate is indicated for every scenario in the book.

Each chapter starts by setting out the focus of the scenarios within, and provides key references and learning outcomes that you should aim to achieve by the end of the chapter. Each scenario reads like a task at an OSCE station, which we recommend you attempt yourself before reading the feedback given for each station.

Before you start tackling the OSCE scenarios, we recommend you first polish your consultation and communication skills by reading this next section.

Consultation/communication skills

This section focuses on the structure of the consultation and the tools that can be used to effectively and efficiently gather information.

Basic structure of the consultation

Ideally the consultation should be patient/client-centred. Accordingly, it should comprise the following five key steps (Das, 2011):

1. Initial open question(s)
2. Targeted history with 'red flags' ('Red flags' are signs or symptoms that warrant referral or urgent action because they suggest significant pathology.)
3. Explore the patient's thoughts and reach a shared understanding
4. Explain the management options and the shared management plan
5. Safety-netting and arranging follow-up, if appropriate.

Initial open question(s)

There are a number of mnemonics that can be used to guide your information-gathering/history-taking (Table 1). Patients should be encouraged to describe their illness in their own words by making optimum use of open questions and facilitation techniques. Try to avoid large numbers of closed questions

Table 1 Mnemonics used to guide information-gathering

O – other people affected/ other symptoms P – provocative and palliative Q – quality and quantity R – region, radiation and recurrence S – severity of symptoms/other symptoms T – timing and treatment U – what do you (the patient) think is wrong	S – site and radiation Q – quality I – intensity T – timing A – aggravating factors R – relieving factors S – secondary symptoms
S – site O – onset (sudden/gradual) C – character (for example dull/sharp/stabbing) R – radiation (of pain) A – associated symptoms T – time course/duration E – exacerbating and relieving factors S – severity	S – site or location I – intensity or severity T – type or nature D – duration O – onset W – with (other symptoms) N – annoyed or aggravated S – spread or radiation I – incidence or frequency pattern R – relieved by
W – who is the patient W – what are the symptoms H – how long have the symptoms been present A – action taken M – medication being taken	A – age/appearance S – self or someone else? M – medication E – extra medicines T – time persisting H – history O – other symptoms D – danger symptoms

asked in a set order. Hastings and Redsell (2006) use the helpful metaphor of someone sorting post into pigeon-holes to explain how to use a mnemonic: 'I let the patient tell me about the problem and as the information is given I slot it into the appropriate place'.

After greeting the patient and introducing yourself, you should encourage the patient to expand on the presenting problem/complaint. To do this you should:

- use open questions (see Box 1) (e.g. 'Tell me about your headaches')
- listen attentively by:

  - looking interested (lean slightly forward and look at patient's face, maintain good eye contact)
  - allowing patients to complete statements without interruption and leave space for patients to think before answering or going on after pausing – give the patient space to talk

- facilitate patients' responses verbally and non-verbally.

Facilitation techniques encourage the patient to speak through verbal and non-verbal means, without directing the

---

Box 1   Open questions

Open questions:

- can be answered in a number of ways
- leave the response open to respondent
- give the respondent a higher degree of freedom
- require more than one or two words
- allow the respondent to express opinions, attitudes, thoughts or feelings
- may encourage the respondent to reveal information which the questioner has not anticipated
- may give you a better idea of a patient's problem and how the patient perceives it.

patient. They indicate to the patient that you are interested in his or her story and include the following tools: probes, pauses/silence, paraphrasing and reflection (see Box 2). If patients are allowed to talk, they usually provide lots of information by themselves. You can then place this information in the appropriate (mental) pigeonhole.

Box 2 Facilitation techniques

Probes
These include:

- questions designed to encourage respondents to expand upon initial responses
- 'follow-up' questions.

    There are several types, including:

- non-verbal probes – a practitioner can indicate a desire for more information by raising or lowering his or her eyebrows, uttering vocalisations such as 'Uh-huh', 'Yes', 'Go on', 'and ... ', 'I see'
- extension probes – 'That's interesting, tell me more?' 'And then what happened?'
- echo probes – involves simply repeating in an inquisitive fashion the last few words uttered by the patient. Patient: 'I've had this pain for a week now'. Practitioner: 'A week?'

Pausing/silence

- Silent periods may make us feel uncomfortable and tempt us to rush in with another question. You should try to resist this.
- Silence/pausing after a question stimulates a response from the patient and helps to prevent you from asking multiple questions.
- Silence/pausing following an initial response from a patient encourages the patient to continue talking (i.e. facilitation).

Paraphrasing

- This is restating in your own words what you heard the patient say.

- It focuses on content (not feelings – cf. reflecting). Patient: 'The headaches started about four weeks ago, I suppose.' Practitioner: 'So you've been having the headaches for about a month.'

Reflecting

- This is mirroring back to patient, in verbal statements, the feeling he or she is communicating.

- You must listen to words about feelings. Patient: 'I've got this terrible cough; it's really starting to get me down.' Practitioner: 'Yes I can see you are upset.'

Training information is provided to the simulated patient you will encounter on the OSCE in order for them to learn to play the part effectively. This might include something like the following: 'If the student starts the consultation with an open question, e.g. "Tell me about the problem" and uses appropriate facilitation techniques, you should reveal further items of the scripted information.'

Targeted history and red flags

This part of the consultation is concerned with building a clearer picture of the presenting problem/complaint by following up on what the patient has already told you with systematic and structured enquiry, in other words, moving from open to targeted closed questions in order to fill the empty pigeonholes (see Box 3). The mnemonics referred to in Table 1 may be used to assist you in doing this. The important thing to remember is that history-taking is most effective when it is discriminating, and each question being asked has a purpose. Mnemonics are a useful starting point to gather information, but additional questioning may be necessary to support decision-making.

> **Box 3**   Closed questions
>
> In closed questions the respondent has no choice in his or her response other than those provided by the questioner. There are three main types:
>
> - selection questions – 'Is the pain dull or throbbing?'
> - yes/no questions – 'Have you got a cough?'
> - identification questions – 'What colour is the phlegm?'
>
>   Closed questions:
>
> - can be answered in one or very few words
> - are restrictive in nature – limited response obtained
> - extract information rapidly and give the questioner high degree of control over the interaction.
>
>   If used too much, closed questions lead to a practitioner-centred consultation. This can result in inaccurate information being obtained and should be avoided.

When using targeted (closed) questions, you should:

- use concise, easily understood questions
- avoid or explain jargon
- avoid using ineffective questions, such as leading, multiple and vague questions; these are unlikely to generate accurate information (see Box 4).

> **Box 4**   Ineffective question types
>
> *Leading questions*
> These lead the respondent towards an expected response. They include:
>
> - simple questions that exert pressure on the patient to acquiesce to the practitioner's point of view: 'You're all right, aren't you?'

- subtle questions that are not immediately obvious as a leading question but worded in such a way as to elicit a certain type of response: 'Do you get headaches frequently, and if so, how often?' 'Do you get headaches occasionally, and if so, how often?'

Leading questions should only be used cautiously since they may put patients in a defensive position, increasing the risk of inaccurate information. The two examples of subtle leading questions above have been shown to result in an over-estimation and underestimation of headaches, respectively.

Multiple questions

These are made up of two or more questions phrased as one: 'Do you cough up any phlegm and is it yellow and have you tried anything for it?' Multiple questions are wasteful and confusing.

Vague questions

These leave the patient unsure how to answer: 'Have you had the pain for quite a while?'

In response to your questions you should always clarify any statements from the patient that are vague or need amplification. For example:

- 'What exactly do you mean by indigestion?'
- 'Can you describe it?'

When in doubt, you should always check the information you are gathering. This may take the form of:

- paraphrasing (see Box 2)
- summarising (see Box 5).

Throughout the information-gathering part of the consultation you should try to pick up verbal and non-verbal cues from the patient (i.e. body language, speech, facial expression), and check out and acknowledge as appropriate. Cues are things that the patient says or does that you do not

---

Box 5 Summarising

Summarising is:

- a brief restatement of the main content and feelings of the interview
- a check back on accuracy: 'Let me check to see if I understand what you have told me so far'.

 It reviews data, identifies what more is needed, checks accuracy, allows the patient to clarify, indicates you are listening and ends the interview.

---

understand, or make you unsure why they mentioned it. They are nearly always hiding important and relevant information:

- 'I've got this terrible cold that's going around, and what with my test and everything I thought I'd better get something for it' [Patient]
- 'You mentioned a test ... ?' [Pharmacist]
- 'Well, you see I've got my driving test in a couple of days and ... ' [Patient]

 Closed questions can also help you identify 'red flags'. 'Red flags' are signs or symptoms that warrant referral or urgent action because they suggest significant pathology. They should not be missed or neglected. Examples include haemoptysis (coughing up of blood) in a patient who presents with cough; difficulty swallowing in a patient presenting with dyspepsia; and visual disturbances associated with a headache.

Explore the patient's thoughts and reach a shared understanding

In this part of the consultation you need to translate your understanding of something into words and concepts patients will understand. This involves taking the patient's existing understanding and moving it towards your understanding (i.e. reaching a shared understanding).

During the information-gathering part of the consultation you will generate your own ideas (e.g. likely cause of
the patient's problem/symptom), concerns (e.g. patient has
red flags) and expectations (e.g. patient will get better without needing any medication). It is also important for you to
recognise that the patient is likely to have come to the pharmacy with her or his own ideas about their problem, which
will have been informed by past experience, discussion with
friends and/or relatives, reading articles in the newspaper or
magazines, the Internet or television (lay referral). They may
have concerns about the problem and almost certainly will
have definite expectations about what they want from you
(the pharmacist). Sometimes the expectations of the patient
will be clear very early on in the consultation (e.g. they have
got a cough and want a cough suppressant); at other times
you may need to actively explore this with the patient. The
key is to recognise the importance of exploring the patient's
ideas, concerns and expectations in order for you to know
the patient's perspective and to achieve a true, shared understanding. Without this, patients are less likely to accept and
follow your advice and management plan. For example, a
patient who comes to the pharmacy with a cough and expects
to get a cough medicine and whose cough you attribute to
being a side-effect of an ACE inhibitor is unlikely to accept
your referral to her GP unless you are able to reach a shared
understanding of the problem.

Explain the management options and the shared management plan

At some stage of most consultations you will need to give
information to patients, such as explaining the management
options and plan, and how to take or use prescribed medication.

Explaining is probably the most difficult of the communication tasks. It involves:

- deciding what information to give the patient – the
  content
- how to give the information – the process.

All too often there is a tendency when explaining to focus on the former – the content – rather than on the latter – the process. There are three essential stages to explaining (see Box 6):

- planning
- presenting
- checking understanding.

Box 6   The three stages to explaining

1. Planning – the content

In most consultations you will need to give information to patients. For example, you may need to explain:

- your assessment of a patient's problem – what's wrong with them
- what you expect to happen and what they should do if it does not
- the management options and plan
- the expected outcome of the management plan
- the safe and effective use of medication.

Planning is crucial to effective explaining and involves deciding how much and the type of information to provide. There are three steps which are important when planning an explanation:

- decide WHAT you are going to explain
- pick out the KEY POINTS around which you are going to build your explanation. These should be kept to the minimum necessary (as far as possible to not more than four, as more are likely to be forgotten)
- work from the KNOWN TO THE UNKNOWN – this point is frequently overlooked and much time is spent explaining things to people who already know or by talking 'over their heads'. Whenever possible you should always find out as much as possible about what the patient already knows.

In other words planning 'good explanations' must take into consideration:

- what is to be explained
- the knowledge of the patient.

To do this you need to find out what the patient:

- knows (e.g. 'I don't know how much you know about benzoyl peroxide and how to use it already.' 'It would be helpful to me to understand a little of what you already know so that I can try to fill any gaps for you')
- would like to know.

Research suggests that, in general, patients want more information. Around 80% are seekers of information and around 20% are avoiders of information. You need to ask the patient what he or she would like to know (e.g. 'There's a lot more information that I'd be happy to share with you about migraine and the drugs used to treat it. Some patients like to know a lot and some prefer to keep it to a minimum. How much information would you like?').

Where there is a lot of information to provide to the patient, it is helpful to give information in small chunks (of no more than four key points). Then pause and check for understanding before proceeding. This is often referred to as 'chunking and checking'.

2. Presentation – the process

Studies of patients' recall of their doctors' and pharmacists' explanations suggest that only a very small portion of the delivered information is retained. Building the following educational strategies into your presentation will help your patient understand and remember essential information.

- *Set aside enough time.* Time is a precious commodity for the pharmacist and the patient. However, an explanation that is hurried is likely to be ineffective. Therefore, set aside enough time.
- *Keep the message simple and brief.* Complexity in an explanation makes for greater difficulty in understanding it. The tendency will be to take in only parts of the explanation, and this can be a recipe for disaster. Explanation should

therefore be kept simple. Brevity is essential so that patients can easily recall and understand the explanation given.

■ *Be clear and fluent*. Clear explanations use appropriate language and are specific. The message must contain language appropriate to the intellectual capacity of the listener and not loaded with jargon. If you must use technical terms, explain their meaning. The message should also be specific, avoiding vague words (e.g 'Drink plenty of water') and expressions. Pace your explanation. It should be fluent and contain pauses. It is annoying and distracting listening to garbled, rambling sentences. Furthermore, lack of fluency in speech may be interpreted by a patient as a lack of knowledge. Lack of fluency is often caused by trying to put too many ideas or facts across in a single sentence and by inadequate planning. Plan your explanation and use sentences that are short and to the point, with pauses in between them. Try to mark out key parts or stages of your explanation (chunking) with short pauses. In short – avoid saying too much, too quickly. Pausing not only enhances understanding, it also allows you time to collect and organise your thoughts.

■ *Focus on the key points*. You should base your explanation on realistic expectations of what your patient can adequately comprehend, depending on his or her previous knowledge and intellectual background, the complexity of the material and the time available. To cover a few essentials well – as far as possible keeping to not more than four key points as more are likely to be forgotten – is a reasonable and honourable goal for most expositions. When you do present a large amount of information, lead off with the key points, since your initial message is often best retained. Pharmacists often explain something better the second time round because the first time they are not sure what the key points are. Often they have not consciously sought them out.

■ *Categorise information*. This is especially useful when you are trying to communicate a complex message. It helps the patient to organise new knowledge and remember it. Categorisation involves telling the patient what categories of information are to be provided, then present the information category by category. For example: 'Now I am going to tell you:

- how omeprazole works;
- what its side-effects are;
- what drugs interact with it;
- how it should be taken.

First, how it works – omeprazole reduces the amount of acid in your stomach', and so on.

- *Summarise information.* Having identified the key points of an explanation, it is important to bring them together in the form of a summary. Summaries are essential for effective explaining. Emphasis breaks up a bland, monotonous explanation. It directs the listener's attention to the most important or essential information. Furthermore, items at the beginning and end of an explanation are more likely to be remembered than items in the middle, so the latter will need to be given emphasis. Important points can be emphasised both verbally and non-verbally. Emphasis can be attached to important items of information verbally using markers – verbal cueing. Markers precede the part of the message which is being emphasised. They may take the form of sequence markers (e.g. 'first', 'second', 'third') or importance markers (e.g. 'this is really important'). Non-verbal emphasis is added to an explanation through change in volume and tone (para-linguistics) and via gestures and movement (body language). Repeat and emphasise key points. The repetition of key items of information helps in the acquisition and retention of knowledge. It is particularly helpful in patient education.

- *Be encouraging.* Patients learn better when they are given praise. Recognise their strengths and acknowledge their efforts. Be enthusiastic.

- *Make an effective conclusion.* Your explanation should also come to an effective conclusion. Choose a few key points to repeat and emphasise (e.g. 'So just to recap – make sure that you use separate face cloth and towel, put one drop into each eye every 2 hours for the next 2 days and then every 4 hours for a further 5 days, and come back and see me if things don't start to improve in 5 days or if they get worse'). You should also ask the patient if there is any other information they would like (e.g. 'Are there any other questions you would like me to answer or any points I haven't covered?'). The conclusion is also the time for a brief message that motivates the patient (e.g. 'I hope that you are feeling better soon').

3. Checking understanding

The third feature of effective explaining is to obtain feedback on whether your explanation has been adequately understood. It is the checking back on understanding that some pharmacists find most difficult.

There are a number of ways of checking that your explanation has been understood:

- You may observe the patient's non-verbal behaviour. Note the raised eyebrows or blank looks.
- Other ways of checking understanding include asking questions, and asking the patient to summarise the explanation.

Safety-netting and arranging follow-up, where appropriate

This is an important component of most consultations, providing protection for both the patient and healthcare practitioner and is essential in all consultations where you are working with limited information (e.g. responding to symptoms). It is also a very useful way of concluding a consultation.

An effective three-part safety net is to explain to the patient:

- what you think the problem is and what you expect to happen (e.g. 'I think the diarrhoea is likely to be caused by an infection and it should clearup by the weekend')
- how he or she would know if you are wrong (e.g. 'If your cold goes on longer than a week or you start to feel worse or start coughing up phlegm which is green or yellow in colour')
- what they should do then (e.g. 'Go and see your doctor').

Occasionally you may wish to arrange follow-up, where appropriate (e.g. 'Come back and see me in six weeks so we can see how your acne is doing').

Now that you have read the introduction, and fresh from advice on consultation and communication skills, you will find scenarios that involve these skills in Chapters 1 and 2.

References and further reading

Charlton R, ed. (2007). *Learning to Consult*. Abingdon: Radcliffe Publishing.

Das TM (2011). *CSA Scenarios for the New MRCGP*, 2nd edn. Banbury: Scion Publishing.

Hastings A, Redsell S, eds (2006). *The Good Consultation Guide for Nurses*. Abingdon: Radcliffe Publishing.

Moulton L (2007). *The Naked Consultation*. Abingdon: Radcliffe Publishing.

Silverman J, Kurtz S, Draper J (2004). *Skills for Communicating with Patients*, 2nd edn. Abingdon: Radcliffe Publishing.

1

Responding to symptoms and history-taking

John Purvis and Cathal Gallagher

Chapter 1 includes scenarios that assess the key skills of responding to symptoms and history-taking. Responding to symptoms is about making decisions (clinical decision-making); it is about deciding what the likely cause of a patient's presenting symptom/complaint might be and how it should be managed.

So what will you need in order to make good decisions when you are confronted with a real or simulated patient who presents with a symptom/complaint?

■ A *good knowledge base* about common diseases (see References and further reading), including their:

  – epidemiology
  – aetiology
  – clinical features
  – prognosis
  – complications
  – management.

OSCE stations that involve responding to symptoms or taking a drug history will often assess your ability to ask appropriate questions, and also to offer information and advice to resolve the problem identified. Knowledge of the typical presenting features of minor ailments and their management will help you handle these scenarios.

- *Analytic and diagnostic reasoning skills.* In order to use your analytic and reasoning skills in the context of responding to symptoms you need to be able to:
  - gather information effectively and efficiently; preferably but not always from the person experiencing the illness/symptom
  - identify and share with the patient the management options and formulate and implement a management plan (this requires effective and efficient information-giving).

- *Consultation/communication skills* (see Introduction).

History-taking is the most important tool when it comes to symptom assessment and diagnosis. The key aims of the history-taking are to:

- get as clear idea of the presenting problem (symptom) as possible
- identify any 'red flags' (signs and symptoms that suggest significant pathology and which therefore require urgent referral)
- identify features that suggest that the likely cause of the presenting problem cannot be appropriately managed by supported self-care and requires referral to another healthcare practitioner (e.g. moderate and severe acne, moderate–severe persistent allergic rhinitis or a drug-induced side-effect).

A systematic approach to history-taking is also included in Chapter 2.

All pharmacists must develop their own way of interacting with members of the public, which reflects their own individual personality. Irrespective of the pharmacist's individual style of history-taking, it is essential that the necessary information is gathered and interpreted before a diagnosis is made. Do not worry if this seems overwhelming at first: the more you practise interacting with the public, the easier it becomes.

In scenarios involving requests for over-the-counter (OTC) medicines, it is essential that you establish some fundamental details, from which to make a diagnosis and recommend a treatment, if appropriate. The 'WWHAM' or 'ASMETHOD' mnemonics will help you to remember these fundamental questions (see Box 1.1). In this chapter, we will concentrate on the WWHAM methodology.

Box 1.1 WWHAM and ASMETHOD mnemonics

WWHAM
- Who is the patient?
- What are the symptoms?
- How long have the symptoms been present?
- Action taken to date
- Medication being taken

ASMETHOD
- Age/appearance
- Self or someone else?
- Medication
- Extra medicines
- Time persisting
- History
- Other symptoms
- Danger symptoms

Key references

Addison B, Brown A, Edwards R, Gray G (2012). *Minor Illness or Major Disease?* 5th edn. London: Pharmaceutical Press.

Blenkinsopp A, Paxton P, Blenkinsopp J (2009). *Symptoms in the Pharmacy: A Guide to the Management of Common Illness*, 6th edn. Oxford: Wiley-Blackwell.

Learning objectives

The following OSCE scenarios assess responding to symptoms and history-taking skills. By the end of this chapter you should be able to:

- use a structured approach to questioning in response to patients' queries regarding signs and symptoms
- offer appropriate advice and information to tackle minor ailments
- refer patients, where appropriate, to other healthcare practitioners
- communicate effectively with patients regarding treatment options.

For each of the following scenarios, remember to read the scenarios fully and consider the topic before starting your interaction with the patient. If you have not already done so, read the section called 'Preparing for OSCE' in the Introduction.

You should not become preoccupied with the specific details of each particular case as you work through these scenarios. These are examples only, and no two patient consultations will ever be identical in practice. Rather, you should concentrate on developing a structured framework for history-taking in general, which you can combine on an ad hoc basis with the knowledge that you have acquired through study of the key references. The scenarios consider the diagnosis and management of a range of symptoms that people may present with in a community pharmacy, including drug-induced side-effects.

Scenario 1.1 Nasal symptoms

Format: Interactive station (encounter with simulated patient)

Supporting material available to student: *BNF*

Time allowed: 5 minutes

Suggested years of study: Undergraduate year 4; pre-registration; postgraduate.

Knowledge and skills tested

- Information-gathering – content and process
- Clinical decision-making/symptom assessment.

Task

It is a Friday afternoon in early January. You are asked to interview a man who is complaining of a blocked nose and feeling really unwell. He is not known to you. Please take a history and attempt to make an assessment of the probable cause of his problem (diagnosis); in the examination situation you might be asked by the examiner what your assessment of the patient's problem is.

- How would you proceed?

Before reading the notes below, you might like to reflect on the key steps of the response to symptoms consultation, in particular:

- the initial open question(s)
- the targeted history with red flags
- exploration of the patient's thoughts and reaching a shared understanding.

If you carry out these stages effectively, the patient/simulated patient should give you the following information:

- He is a man in his early forties.
- He has a blocked nose and feels really unwell.
- His cold started 5 days ago with the following symptoms:
  - blocked nose – both sides
  - nasal discharge – watery at first then thick and yellow
  - sneezing
  - scratchy throat
  - dry (unproductive) cough.

- He currently feels shivery and sweaty but he has not taken his temperature.
- He feels really washed-out.
- He has a feeling of fullness in the face.
- He has a dull pain behind his right cheek, which is made worse when he bends down.
- His nose is still blocked and he has a greenish yellow thick nasal discharge.
- He has tried some Sudafed® (pseudoephedrine) tablets but they have not helped.
- He has not used any nose drops or spray.
- He is not taking any medication for any other medical condition(s).

Scenario 1.1 feedback

When confronted with this presentation (blocked nose) you should:

- take a history
- initially establish if both sides or only one side of the nose are affected – bilateral or unilateral nasal obstruction.

Bilateral or unilateral?

- Bilateral obstruction is common and occurs in conditions associated with mucosal oedema (e.g. upper respiratory tract infection, allergic and non-allergic rhinitis).
- Nasal obstruction may be asymmetrical – due to nasal cycle.
- Unilateral obstruction is rare and occurs in conditions associated with abnormal anatomy or mass.
- If unilateral, refer patient to her or his GP.
- If bilateral, you should determine if:
  - it is a new event
  - it is chronic or recurrent
  - there are any other associated symptoms/clinical features.

Is it a new event?

- It has been present for no more than a few days.
- Most likely diagnosis is upper respiratory tract infection (URTI).
- Check for other clinical features of URTI.
- The common cold may be associated with:
  - sneezing
  - postnasal discharge – cough/throat clearing
  - sore throat
  - headache
  - fever
  - hoarseness
  - malaise.

- In acute sinusitis there may be two phases to the illness, often referred to as double sickness or double worsening: symptoms of viral URTI worse at day 2, then better, then worse a few (3–5) days later.
- Other features of acute sinusitis may include:
  - coloured/purulent nasal discharge
  - facial pain/headache
  - maxillary toothache.

Is it chronic or recurrent?

- Is it present continuously or intermittently for more than, say, three weeks?
- Is it seasonal? In which case, the diagnosis is almost certainly seasonal allergic rhinitis – hay fever.
- Check for other clinical features of seasonal allergic rhinitis, such as:
  - serial sneezing
  - nasal itching
  - ocular irritation
  - itching of soft palate
  - itching in ear canal.

- If not seasonal, it may be:
  - perennial allergic rhinitis
  - vasomotor rhinitis

- rhinitis medicamentosis or
- drug-induced rhinitis.

■ Try to determine timing of symptoms and any triggers.

Timing
■ In perennial allergic rhinitis, symptoms may:
  - be nocturnal – house dust mite allergy
  - occur after certain household activities (e.g. bed making) – house dust mite allergy.

■ Vasomotor rhinitis symptoms may occur monthly.

Triggers
■ In perennial allergic rhinitis, triggers include:
  - house dust
  - contact with animals, especially cats.

■ In vasomotor rhinitis, triggers can be:

  - stress – excess parasympathetic activity
  - hormonal changes (e.g. menstruation, pregnancy, oral contraceptives)
  - environmental factors, such as marked temperature changes, barometric pressure changes, bright lights
  - chemical irritants (e.g. perfumes, sprays)
  - alcohol
  - spicy foods.

■ In rhinitis medicamentosis, persistent use of over-the-counter topical nasal decongestants (or cocaine) may act as a trigger.
■ Drug-induced rhinitis may be caused by a number of drugs, including:

  - ACE inhibitors
  - beta blockers, especially topical ocular preparations used to treat glaucoma
  - chlorpromazine
  - aspirin and NSAIDs (non-steroidal anti-inflammatory drugs)

- methyldopa
- prazosin
- oral contraceptives.

Look for 'red flags'

- Unilateral nasal obstruction (blocked nose) – may suggest mass.
- Unilateral nasal discharge, especially if purulent and/or bloody, and especially in elderly – may suggest malignancy.
- Double worsening (symptoms worse at day 2, then better, then worse a few days later) – may suggest acute sinusitis.
- Prolonged use of topical nasal decongestants.

Probable cause of patient's presenting problem/symptom

Acute sinusitis.

Suggested revision points

- Clinical features and management of sinusitis.

Scenario 1.2 Eye symptoms

Format: Interactive station (encounter with simulated patient)

Supporting material available to student: *BNF*

Time allowed: 5 minutes

Suggested years of study: Undergraduate year 4; pre-registration; postgraduate.

Knowledge and skills tested

- Information-gathering – content and process
- Clinical decision-making/symptom assessment.

Task

It is Monday morning. You are asked to interview a woman who is complaining of a sore eye. She is not known to you. Please take a history and observe the affected eye(s) and attempt to make an assessment of the probable cause of her problem (diagnosis). In the examination situation you might be asked by the examiner what your assessment of the patient's problem is.

■   How would you proceed?

Before reading the notes below, you might like to reflect on the key steps of the response to symptoms consultation, in particular:

■   the initial open question(s)
■   the targeted history with red flags
■   exploration of the patient's thoughts and reaching a shared understanding.

If you carry out these stages effectively the patient/simulated patient should give you the following information:

■   She is a woman in her thirties.
■   Her right eye started feeling 'scratchy' yesterday but both eyes are affected now, although the discomfort experienced by her right eye is greater.
■   She describes the discomfort as scratchy/grittiness of the surface of her eyes – she has no pain in or around the eye.
■   Her eyelids were stuck together when she woke up this morning and she had to bathe them to open them.
■   There was dried crusty material at the base of her eyelashes.
■   She has a discharge from both eyes which is quite thick and contains some yellowish matter.
■   She has experienced no problems with her vision.
■   She has not experienced any discomfort in bright light (photophobia).
■   She has no other symptoms.

- Her symptoms began shortly after her son was sent home from school with 'red eye'.
- She does not wear contact lenses.
- She is not currently taking or using any medication.

If you asked to observe/examine the eye(s) the patient would have shown you a photograph, from which you would/should have noticed the following:

- that both eyes are infected/red – right more so than left eye
- that the redness is most marked in fornix and angles
- that there is no ciliary flush
- that the cornea looks bright and healthy
- that both pupils appear round and the same size.

Scenario 1.2 feedback

You need to gather subjective (history) and objective (observation) information. Initially you should find out if:

- both eyes or only one eye are/is affected – bilateral or unilateral?
- there is associated pain
- there is a discharge and if so what is it like – watery, mucopurulent, and does it cause stickiness/crusting (eyelashes slightly matted together on awakening in the morning)?

The information gained helps narrow down the cause/diagnosis.

Other subjective information (from history), which will help identify the cause includes:

- time of onset
- any previous episodes

- associated symptoms, including discomfort/itching, and if so its location and nature (e.g. gritty, burning), photophobia, visual change, haloes (colours around bright lights), loss of vision, upper respiratory tract symptoms – often seen with viral and allergic conjunctivitis
- history of atopy/allergy
- contact with individuals with similar problems
- use of medication – ocular.

Objective information (from examination) you should gather, which will help identify the cause/red flags, includes:

- pattern of redness – is it generalised, localised, circumcorneal (ciliary flush)? (Unilateral red eye suggests causes other than conjunctivitis.)
- does the cornea appear bright or cloudy?
- size and shape of the pupil – should be circular, central and equal in size (look for irregularity and inequality in size)
- pain
- true (consensual) photophobia (when shining a light into the unaffected eye causes pain in the affected eye when the affected eye is shut/closed)
- poor vision/loss of vision
- pus in the cornea or anterior chamber as opposed to mucopurulent discharge associated with bacterial conjunctivitis
- pupil abnormality – such as abnormal size or shape, or poor constriction to light
- coloured haloes around point of light in the patient's vision
- acid or alkali burns.

Probable cause of patient's presenting problem/symptom

Acute bacterial conjunctivitis.

Suggested revision points

- Eye structure and function
- Management of bacterial conjunctivitis, including over-the-counter options
- How to use eye drops (see also Scenario 7.6).

Scenario 1.3 Dry cough

Format: Interactive station (encounter with simulated patient)

Supporting material: *BNF*

Time allowed: 5 minutes

Suggested years of study: Undergraduate years 1–4; pre-registration.

Knowledge and skills tested

- Application of a structured framework for assessment of symptoms
- Management of minor ailments
- Communication skills.

Task

A customer enters your pharmacy and wishes to speak to you. The customer tells you that they 'need something for a cough'. Using a structured approach to symptom assessment, question the customer and decide upon an appropriate course of action.

- What questions should you ask?
- What advice would you give?

By asking the appropriate questions, you should obtain the necessary information to either refer or treat the patient. For example, the patient may tell you that he or she:

- has a dry persistent cough
- is not bringing up any phlegm
- does not have a cold, sore throat or any other viral symptoms
- has had the symptoms for the last three weeks
- has been taking ramipril tablets 5 mg daily for the past six weeks, for newly diagnosed hypertension.

Scenario 1.3 feedback

What questions would you ask?

1. Establish who is the patient (*Who?*). Are you talking to the patient or their representative? How old is the patient? Are they male or female?
2. Ask what symptoms are being experienced by the patient (*What?*). At this stage, be mindful of the broadest differences in possible diagnoses (Is the cough dry or productive?), and try to refine your opinion with each follow-on question (Is there any nasal congestion/chest pain/coloured or foul-smelling sputum associated with the productive cough?) until you arrive at some likely candidate diagnoses.
3. Establish the duration of the symptoms (*How long?*). This may indicate the need for referral.
4. Ask if any treatments have already been tried (*Any action?*). Consider this not only from the perspective of ruling out treatments that have not been effective, but also from the viewpoint of trying to ascertain whether the existing treatment has aggravated the condition (cough suppressants are not beneficial in cases of productive cough).
5. Ask whether the patient takes any medicines for other medical conditions (*Medications?*). Refer back to your accumulated knowledge base. Can any medications cause a cough of the type the patient describes?

In this scenario the WWHAM mnemonic will give you the minimum required information, but don't forget that other mnemonics can help you dig further into the history.

On identifying the cause of the problem you should then offer advice and, if appropriate, recommend OTC medication to treat the problem. In this scenario you should:

- offer advice on symptomatic relief of the cough
- advise the patient that the symptoms may be caused by the new medication, ramipril, and that this may need to be reviewed by his or her GP.

Suggested revision points

- Structured frameworks for responding to symptoms
- ACE inhibitor side-effects.

Scenario 1.4 Diarrhoea

Format: Interactive station (encounter with simulated patient)

Supporting material available to student: *BNF*

Time allowed: 5 minutes

Suggested years of study: Undergraduate year 4; pre-registration; postgraduate.

Knowledge and skills tested

- Information-gathering – content and process
- Clinical decision-making/symptom assessment.

Task

It is Monday morning. You are asked to interview a man who is complaining of diarrhoea. He is not known to you. Please take a history and attempt to make an assessment of the probable cause of his problem (diagnosis). In the examination situation you might be asked by the examiner what your assessment of the patient's problem is.

- How would you proceed?

Before reading the notes below, you might like to reflect on the key steps of the response to symptoms consultation, in particular:

- the initial open question(s)
- the targeted history with red flags
- exploration of the patient's thoughts and reaching a shared understanding.

If you carry out these stages effectively the patient/simulated patient should give you the following information:

- He is experiencing diarrhoea.
- He is 32 years old.
- He has had diarrhoea for the past 24 hours.
- The diarrhoea came on suddenly.
- He is passing watery stools.
- He is also experiencing mild cramping abdominal pain poorly localised around the navel.
- He felt sick before the diarrhoea started but has not vomited.
- He feels generally off-colour but has not had a fever, chills or night sweats.
- He has not seen any blood in the stools.
- He has had to empty his bowels six to eight times in the last 24-hour period.
- He last went to the toilet about an hour before coming to the pharmacy.
- He has not been in contact with anyone who has had diarrhoea.
- He has not recently travelled abroad.
- He completed a course of amoxicillin (500 mg three times a day for 5 days) for a chest infection 2 days ago.
- He is not taking any other prescribed medicines.
- He has an important meeting at work tomorrow.

Scenario 1.4 feedback – the clinical approach

When confronted with someone reporting diarrhoea you should first confirm that it is the man who is experiencing diarrhoea. Then you should determine whether:

- the patient actually has diarrhoea (to do this you need to determine what the patient means by diarrhoea in terms of stool frequency and nature of the stools)
- the diarrhoea is acute, intermittent or chronic (if acute, find out whether there are any clues to an infectious cause, such as contact with other affected individuals, a group of people affected who have eaten a common meal or recent return from abroad (red flag))
- there are additional symptoms, including nausea and vomiting, abdominal pain, fever (red flag)
- the patient is taking any medication – a wide range of drugs may be associated with diarrhoea, including antibiotics (especially ampicillin, amoxicillin, second-generation cephalosporins, clindamycin), alcohol, alpha-glucosidase inhibitors, laxatives, magnesium-containing antacids, selective serotonin reuptake inhibitors (SSRIs)
- there has been blood in the stool (red flag) – the presence of blood in the stools of a patient with acute diarrhoea raises the probability of bacterial gastroenteritis (which is notifiable); however, it is important to note that inflammatory bowel disease can present as acute attacks of bloody diarrhoea (a history of previous attacks will usually be found)
- the patient is dehydrated – most acute diarrhoea is caused by self-limiting infection (usually viral) with dehydration being the most important complication. Any patient showing signs and symptoms of dehydration must be referred urgently for medical assessment and management (red flag). Infants and the elderly people are particularly susceptible to the effects of dehydration.

Other red flags not listed above are chronic diarrhoea and weight loss associated with chronic diarrhoea.

Probable cause of patient's presenting problem/symptom

■ Medication-related (antibiotic-associated) diarrhoea – most likely; or viral diarrhoea.

Suggested revision points

■ Causes and management of diarrhoea.

Scenario 1.5 Rash

> Format: Interactive station (encounter with simulated patient)
>
> Supporting material: *BNF*
>
> Time allowed: 5 minutes
>
> Suggested years of study: Undergraduate years 1–4; pre-registration.

Knowledge and skills tested

■ Application of a structured framework for symptom assessment
■ Management of minor ailments
■ Communication skills.

Task

A customer enters your pharmacy and asks you for something to treat a rash on both their hands. Speak to the customer in order to assess the presenting problem, and give appropriate advice.

■ What questions do you ask?
■ What advice do you give? (Read the notes below after listing the questions you would ask.)

If you ask the appropriate questions, the patient may tell you that:

- the symptoms began 2 days ago and the hands are getting more itchy and sore (the area looks red and angry)
- it's never happened before and the patient has not had eczema or any other skin condition before this
- the patient has not eaten anything out of the ordinary
- the patient has been using a new dishwashing liquid
- the patient has tried calamine lotion but it is not helping
- the patient has not taken any oral antihistamines
- there are no other symptoms
- the patient is asthmatic and uses a salbutamol inhaler
- the patient is allergic to penicillin.

Scenario 1.5 feedback

What questions would you ask?

1. Establish who the patient is (*Who?*).
2. Ask what symptoms are being experienced by the patient (*What?*). Are there any trigger factors (i.e. does the patient think they have done something that may have caused the symptoms: new washing-up detergent, soap, gloves)? Having established the cause, you can then offer appropriate advice on how to treat the symptoms and reduce the risk of the same problem recurring.
3. Establish the duration of the symptoms (*How long?*).
4. Ask if any treatments have already been tried (*Action?*).
5. Ask whether the patient takes any medicines for other medical conditions (*Medications?*). Consider this in conjunction with question 2: allergic reactions to new medications may cause a rash, which will usually appear after a few doses.

What advice do you give?

Once you have established the nature and probable cause of the problem, you should then offer advice regarding

symptomatic relief with appropriate over-the-counter medication. This could include an oral antihistamine if itch is
a particular problem, or short-term use of hydrocortisone
1%, or an emollient. The patient's preference on the type of
medication should be sought. Appropriate advice regarding
how to take or use the medication advised should be offered.
In addition, you should advise the customer to stop using the
dishwashing liquid or to wear gloves (remove the cause), and
advise the customer to see his or her GP if symptoms persist
or worsen.

Suggested revision points

- Structured frameworks for responding to symptoms
- Treatment of minor skin problems in the pharmacy.

Scenario 1.6 Constipation

Format: Interactive station (encounter with simulated
patient)

Supporting material available to student: *BNF*, a range
of laxative preparations in their original packaging containing Patient Information Leaflets

Time allowed: 5 minutes

Suggested years of study: Undergraduate year 4; pre-
registration; postgraduate.

Knowledge and skills tested

- Information-giving – content and process
- Patient management.

Task

It is Monday morning. You have just interviewed a woman
who presented complaining of constipation, which you have

diagnosed/assessed as short duration functional constipation. She is not known to you. Please explain your diagnosis and management plan, in order to reach a shared understanding.

■ How would you proceed?

Before reading the notes below, you might like to reflect on the key steps of the response to symptoms consultation, in particular:

■ explain the management options and implement the shared management plan

■ safety-netting and arranging follow-up, if appropriate.

If you carry out these stages effectively the patient/simulated patient should give you the following information:

■ She is 30 years old.

■ She normally empties her bowels once a day, usually after breakfast.

■ For the past couple of weeks she has only managed to empty her bowels twice a week.

■ She has to strain to pass a motion.

■ She describes her stools as small and hard.

■ She has not noticed any blood in or on the stools.

■ She does not experience any pain when she empties her bowels.

■ She has no other symptoms.

■ She has recently started a new job and the associated change in routine means she no longer allows time to empty her bowels in a morning, indeed she often has to skip breakfast now.

■ Her diet is mostly convenience foods and takeaways – she does not eat much fresh fruit and vegetables and eats white rather than wholemeal bread.

■ She does not take regular exercise.

■ Her daily fluid intake is estimated at about 1.5 litres per day.

■ She has not taken anything for constipation.

■ She is not currently taking any medication.

Scenario 1.6 feedback

You should explain that her constipation is probably caused by a combination of things associated with her lifestyle.

Explain the management options. Treatment is best done by educating the patient. This could include:

- explaining variations in normal bowel habit
- reminding the patient of the need to allow time to defecate and not to 'ignore the call to stool'
- encouraging the patient to exercise regularly according to the individual's abilities and explaining why physical activity is important
- explaining the importance of adequate fluid intake – at least 2 litres – the equivalent of 6–8 tumblers of liquid daily
- explaining the importance of dietary fibre – adults should consume 18–30 g per day, and an increase in intake may take as long as four weeks to have an effect
- explaining that oral laxatives could be used if dietary measures are ineffective, or while waiting for them to take effect.

If you recommend oral laxatives:

- start treatment with a bulk-forming laxative (adequate fluid intake is important)
- if stools remain hard, add or switch to an osmotic laxative
- if stools are soft but the person still finds them difficult to pass or complains of inadequate emptying, add a stimulant laxative
- advise the person that they can be stopped once the stools become soft and easily passed again.

Remember that:

- The use of oral (stimulant and osmotic) laxatives can lead to the development of a vicious cycle: constipation is relieved by the laxative; consequently, the patient has no urge to defecate for several days and perceives that she is constipated again and resumes (or requests more) laxatives. Patients should be appropriately educated to avoid this.

■ It may take several days before bulk laxatives and lactulose have any effect. This should be explained to the patient, since the expectation might be that they would exert an effect more quickly, and the patient may interpret failure to do so as the laxatives not working.

Suggested revision points

■ Drug treatment of constipation including medication counselling points.

Scenario 1.7 Drug history

Format: Written station

Supporting material available to student: e.g. *BNF*

Time allowed: 5 minutes

Suggested years of study: Undergraduate years 3–4; pre-registration; postgraduate.

Knowledge and skills tested

■ Taking a drug history.

Task

You are the pharmacist on a hospital ward. You are approached by a doctor whom you know well. He asks you whether selegiline can cause vertigo. What questions would you ask the doctor before the query can be answered?

You are not expected to state whether the drug causes the side-effect. The purpose of the task is for you to identify what information you need before you are able to find out whether the drug can cause the side-effect.

Scenario 1.7 feedback

To enable you to target your search for information to address the question posed by the doctor, you need to ask questions to establish some information:

- Relevant patient details (e.g. age), as some patients, including the elderly, may be more susceptible to side-effects.
- How long has the patient had the vertigo? Or, when did the vertigo appear in relation to the initiation of selegiline? This question would help you to establish whether there may be a link between starting the treatment and the development of the side-effect.
- Describe the vertigo (signs, symptoms, severity, is it getting better or worse?).
- How long has the patient been taking the selegiline?
- What dose, and for what indication?
- What other medication is the patient taking and at what dose(s), including over-the-counter, herbal or homeopathic medications? This question is asked so that you can ascertain whether there may be other causes for the symptom experienced.
- Has any other medication been started or stopped during this time? Again, this is asked in order to eliminate causes of the symptom.
- Any other pre-existing medical problems/conditions/drug allergies of relevance (that may have caused the vertigo)?
- Has any action already been taken to address the problem?

Suggested revision points

- Sources of information on side-effects of drugs.

Scenario 1.8 Mouth symptoms

Format: Interactive station (encounter with simulated patient)

Supporting material available to student: *BNF*

Time allowed: 5 minutes

Suggested years of study: Undergraduate year 4; preregistration; postgraduate.

Knowledge and skills tested

- Information-gathering – content and process
- Clinical decision-making/symptom assessment.

Task

It is Tuesday afternoon. You are asked to interview a woman who is complaining of a mouth ulcer. She is not known to you. Please take a history and observe the lesion and attempt to make an assessment of the probable cause of her problem (diagnosis). In the examination situation you might be asked by the examiner what your assessment of the patient's problem is.

- How would you proceed?

Before reading the notes below, you might like to reflect on the key steps of the response to symptoms consultation, in particular:

- the initial open question(s)
- the targeted history with red flags
- exploration of the patient's thoughts and reaching a shared understanding.

If you carry out these stages effectively the patient/simulated patient should give you the following information:

- She is 21 years old.
- She is a final-year university student studying history.
- The ulcer is painful.
- She first noticed it this morning.
- She has been bothered by mouth ulcers since she was a child but she has not had one for several months.

- She usually only gets a single ulcer at a time, as on this occasion, but occasionally there may be two or three.
- She often experiences a prickling sensation before the ulcer(s) appears.
- They do not always occur at the same site but always on either the inside of the lips or cheeks.
- They are always similar in size and heal within a couple of weeks.
- She has no other symptoms.
- She is not taking any medication.
- She is currently revising hard for her exams next week and the discomfort is interfering with her revision.

If you asked to observe/examine the patient's mouth, she would have shown you a photograph, from which you would/should have noticed the following:

- There is a single ulcer on the inside of the lower lip (buccal mucosa) close to the buccal sulcus.
- The ulcer is round in shape and about 5 mm in diameter.
- The ulcer is a grey-yellow colour and is surrounded by an erythematous border.

Scenario 1.8 feedback

When a patient presents with a mouth ulcer or sore mouth you should:

- gather information, both subjective (take a history) and objective (have a look/observe)
- determine the age of the patient – viral infections and aphthous stomatitis (ulcers) are more common in children and adolescents.

You should then find out:

- how long the ulcer/ulcers have been present – are they persistent or non-persistent? An individual with an ulcer that persists for more than three weeks without evidence of healing should be referred (red flag)

- whether one or more than one ulcer is present (red flag: a solitary, persistent and often painless ulcer could be malignant)
- whether the ulcer(s) is/are painful – a painless ulcer, especially in an elderly patient, that has been present for several weeks suggests carcinoma
- whether there have been any previous episodes – recurrent vesicles/ulcer on the lips and/or mucocutaneous junction suggest herpes simplex, recurrent ulcers in the mouth suggest aphthous stomatitis (of which there are several types – minor, major and herpetiform)
- where in the mouth the ulcer(s) occur
- the size, shape and colour of ulcers – you will need to look
- if the patient is aware of anything that may have caused the ulcer(s) (particularly likely with traumatic ulcers)
- if any tingling or itching before the ulcer appears – indicates possible herpes simplex, herpes zoster or aphthous stomatitis
- if any extra-oral features are present (e.g. gastrointestinal symptoms, skin lesions) (red flag: associated gastrointestinal symptoms such as diarrhoea, abdominal pain and blood-stained stools with mucus suggests associated inflammatory bowel disease)
- if the patient has recently started any drug therapy.

If the ulcers are recurrent, you also need to find out:

- at what sites in the mouth the ulcers occur
- how long they take to heal
- how many the patient may have at any one time
- whether the patient has had ulcers at any other body sites
- whether the patient is aware of any factors that predispose to ulcers.

In addition to the red flags mentioned above, consider:

- associated ocular inflammation (anterior uveitis) and genital ulceration

- drug treatment: blood dyscrasias are a rare but significant side-effect of some treatments (e.g. gold, carbimazole); oral ulceration may be a first sign.

Probable cause of patient's presenting problem/symptom

Minor aphthous stomatitis/ulcer.

Suggested revision points

- Clinical features of mouth problems that may present in a pharmacy
- Over-the-counter management of mouth problems.

Scenario 1.9 Skin problems

Format: Interactive station (encounter with simulated patient)

Supporting material available to student: *BNF*, a pack of 5% benzoyl peroxide gel/cream, including the PIL (Patient Information Leaflets)

Time allowed: 5 minutes

Suggested years of study: Undergraduate year 4; pre-registration; postgraduate.

Knowledge and skills tested

- Information-giving – content and process
- Medication counselling.

Task

You have just interviewed a young man who presented with spots on his face and have diagnosed the cause as mild acne vulgaris. He has tried Oxy 10® (benzoyl peroxide lotion), which has not helped. You suspect this is because he used it incorrectly. As part of your management plan for his acne you decide to prescribe 5% benzoyl peroxide aqueous gel/cream.

Please explain your diagnosis, management plan – including how to use benzoyl peroxide – and any safety-netting, in order to reach a shared understanding.

Your assessment of the patient is based on the following patient information:

- He is 17 years old.
- He has been pressurised into getting something for his spots by his mother.
- His skin is greasy and he has open comedones (blackheads) and a few inflamed papules on his cheeks and around the chin.
- He does not have any acne lesions anywhere else.
- His spots make him feel dirty.
- He washes his face several (5 or 6) times a day, with normal soap and water.
- He has not used any special cleaning agents.
- He has tried Oxy 10® (benzoyl peroxide 10%), which he says has not really helped and has made his skin sore.
- He applied the Oxy 10® to the individual spots.
- He is concerned that eating fatty foods and chocolate gives you spots – something his mother told him.
- He is not too down about his spots and appears somewhat resigned to the fact that there is nothing that can be done about them.
- You are also supplied with a photograph which shows mild acne vulgaris.

Scenario 1.9 feedback

You should:

- reassure the person and give practical advice on coping with acne
- reassure the person that acne is very common, will not last forever, and treatment is effective

- dispel common myths (acne is not caused by poor diet or hygiene and is not infectious)
- advise on good skin care (skin should not be washed too frequently or vigorously, and spots should not be picked)
- explain that management options include benzoyl peroxide or referral to GP, who can prescribe other treatments
- explain that benzoyl peroxide if used correctly does work in mild acne
- explain that benzoyl peroxide will prevent new spots, not get rid of existing ones; accordingly, it should be applied to all at risk areas, not just to the spots that are present
- choose a suitable strength (2.5% or 5% usually effective and less likely to cause side-effects) and vehicle according to skin type (Gels are useful for oily skin, creams for dry skin, and lotions for application to large areas of skin. Alcoholic applications should be avoided in people with very sensitive skin.)
- explain how to use benzoyl peroxide according to the Patient Information Leaflet you are provided with.

Safety net by:

- explaining that treatment may take several months (at least eight weeks) to work
- encouraging him to return after six weeks (opportunity for you to check on treatment and provide encouragement)
- advising him to see his GP if the condition gets worse – more lesions, painful lesions, other acne-prone areas become involved (chest, back, shoulders).

Suggested revision points

- Diagnosis of skin problems that may present in a community pharmacy
- Management of acne, including medication counselling points.

Scenario 1.10 Throat symptoms

Format: Interactive station (encounter with simulated patient)

Supporting material available to student: e.g. *BNF*

Time allowed: 5 minutes

Suggested years of study: Undergraduate years 1–4; pre-registration; postgraduate.

Knowledge and skills tested

- History-taking
- Application of knowledge identified in the *BNF*.

Task

A customer visiting a community pharmacy wishes to speak to the pharmacist regarding a severe sore throat. You are required to ask the patient regarding their presenting problem, and to offer appropriate advice in relation to the presenting problem.

On questioning, the patient tells you that they:

- have experienced the symptoms for 4 days
- have an overactive thyroid, treated with carbimazole (20 mg twice daily); treatment started 3 weeks ago, initiated by the endocrinologist
- do not take other regular medication
- are also feverish and dizzy
- have been using lozenges for sore throat for the last few days, and taken paracetamol tablets at maximum dosage for 3 days, both to no effect.

Scenario 1.10 feedback

Using the WWHAM framework in this scenario would have enabled you to establish that the patient takes carbimazole for hyperthyroidism. You could then confirm the dose, and duration of therapy. At this point in the interaction it would be appropriate for you to look in the *BNF* to identify the possible side-effects of carbimazole. In the *BNF* you should have found counselling advice to warn patients to report immediately if sore throat, mouth ulcers, bruising, fever, malaise or non-specific illness develop. This is because these signs and symptoms are indicators of bone marrow suppression which is a rare but serious side-effect of carbimazole.

Having established the patient takes carbimazole and no other medication, you should have advised the patient that the problem may be a sign of carbimazole toxicity. Therefore they should be referred to the GP urgently.

Suggested revision points

- Drugs that can cause blood dyscrasias, such as methotrexate and other immunosuppressants.

Chapter 1 feedback summary

In Chapter 1 you have looked at a range of responding to symptoms scenarios and elements of history-taking. You will have learned the importance of effective consultation and communication skills to elicit a history. A reliable history enables you to offer appropriate advice in relation to self-management with or without over-the-counter drugs, and to refer patients to other healthcare professionals where necessary.

Now that you have completed this chapter, assess your competence in the knowledge and skills listed in Table 1.1. Jot down any notes that may help you.

If there are any points that you consider need further work, start a CPD (continuous professional development) cycle now to identify how you can achieve this action.

Table 1.1 Chapter 1 learning outcomes

Knowledge and skills	More work required	Feel competent
Use a structured approach to questioning in response to patients' queries regarding signs and symptoms		
Offer appropriate advice and information to tackle minor ailments		
Refer patients appropriately to other healthcare practitioners		
Communicate effectively with patients regarding treatment options		

References and further reading

Hopcroft K, Forte V (2010). *Symptom Sorter*, 4th edn. Abingdon: Radcliffe Publishing.

Johnson G, Hill-Smith I (2012). *The Minor Illness Manual*, 4th edn. Abingdon: Radcliffe Publishing.

Polmear A, ed. (2008). *Evidence-based Diagnosis in Primary Care*. Oxford: Elsevier.

PRODIGY. http://prodigy.clarity.co.uk/home (accessed 1 October 2012).

Rutter P (2009). *Community Pharmacy*, 2nd edn. Edinburgh: Churchill Livingstone.

Schroeder K (2010). *The 10-Minute Clinical Assessment*. Oxford: Wiley-Blackwell.

2

Systems-based client assessment

Julia Williams, Matthew Catterall,
John Donaghy, Sarah Jardine, Paul Power,
John Talbot and Gary Venstone

Chapter 2 focuses on clinical history-taking and client assessment skills within a community setting. A key aim of this chapter is to help you to differentiate between those clients who can be treated safely at the point of first contact and those who may need to be referred to an alternative care pathway. Client assessment is complex and wide ranging, so this chapter can only introduce you to some of the essential elements of this part of your professional practice.

Before you embark on the following scenarios, take some time to consider your approach to client assessment. Think about the purpose of a systematic clinical history and identify what knowledge you need to have to make best use of the information gained from the client's history in order to make appropriate decisions about client assessment. Some key references are listed at the end of this chapter.

Learning objectives

The following OSCE scenarios assess your knowledge of systematic clinical history-taking, your approach to systems based clinical assessment, and your performance of a variety of clinical skills. By the end of this chapter you should be able to:

- obtain a systematic clinical history from a client
- describe the stages of a clinical examination of the respiratory system

- recognise an emergency cardiac event
- understand reasons for a neurological assessment
- understand how to use a binaural acoustic stethoscope
- understand how to undertake a blood glucose measurement
- understand how to assess a client's pulse and respiration
- formulate a working diagnosis
- offer appropriate advice to clients.

For each of the following scenarios, remember to read the scenarios fully and think about the topic before you begin.

Scenario 2.1 Clinical history

Format: Interactive station

Supporting material available to student: *BNF*, paper to document notes

Time allowed: 10–15 minutes depending on level of study

Suggested years of study: Undergraduate years 1–4; pre-registration; postgraduate.

Knowledge and skills tested

- Obtaining a clinical history from a client
- Formulating a working diagnosis
- Advising the client on a basic management plan.

Task

A 50-year-old man attends the pharmacy for advice on his recent low back pain. Before you can give him advice you need to find out more about his condition. Take a clinical history from him and advise him on the management of his pain.

Think about the questions that you would ask and the reasons for asking them. If the client had been asked the relevant questions he would have told you that he:

■ works in property maintenance and is self-employed
■ hurt his back while lifting a heavy object 2 days ago
■ has pain in his lower back which is central and also slightly to the right
■ feels that the pain is slightly better than it was initially, but feels he would like advice on pain management
■ has had this problem before, and it resolved while being managed with over-the-counter 'pain-killers' and a short time off work
■ has had no bladder or bowel changes
■ has no anaesthesia or paraesthesia either in the saddle area or down the legs
■ is generally fit and well with no unexplained weight loss
■ occasionally uses a salbutamol inhaler for generally well-controlled asthma; no other medications
■ has no allergies.

Scenario 2.1 feedback

At the beginning of this task did you introduce yourself to the client, ask his name and tell him what you wanted to do? It is important that the client knows that you are going to ask several questions in order to help him, so that he can give his consent for you to do this. The client may be expecting you just to prescribe medication for him so may not anticipate the detail of some of the questions you are going to ask him. It is essential that you establish rapport with the client if you want the client to feel comfortable with you so that the subsequent history is useful and accurate.

■ Did you ensure that you were in an environment that was private and without distractions – for you and for him?
■ Did you find out how old the client was? This can have an influence on what you think might be the problem and therefore on the advice you give him.

You should have approached the questioning in a logical and thorough manner. Remember that taking a history from a client involves you listening carefully to the answers, responding and following up on the answers accordingly, not just asking a prearranged list of questions. It is useful to work through the following areas, bearing in mind that, at times, you will adapt this to ensure that your conversation with the client has a natural flow, and that you are able to follow any leads the client may give you.

Presenting complaint (PC)

This is where you clarify what the client has come to see you about. Remember that the first thing he says may not be the main complaint; he may need to relax and work his way round to discussing the key issue(s). Make sure that you fully understand what he has said about the presenting complaint before you move on to other elements of the history.

History of presenting complaint (HPC)

This is when you find out the specific details of the problem. How long has he had the pain? What was he doing when it came on? Did it come on suddenly or gradually? Where exactly is the pain and does it go anywhere else (radiate)? Is it there all the time? Is he getting any other symptoms, such as anaesthesia (numbness) or paraesthesia (pins and needles)? How bad is the pain (perhaps use a pain scale from 1 to 10, with 10 being the worst pain he has ever experienced)? Does the level of pain fluctuate? Has it changed since onset? What makes the pain worse? What makes the pain better? Is he able to sleep at night? If so, in what position? What has he done since the pain came on (activity/work and treatment)? There will be other questions you will ask your client depending on what he tells you.

It is important to ask about 'red flag' symptoms (meaning symptoms that should not be ignored and require urgent medical advice), which would lead you to be concerned that the pain may be more complicated or sinister than it first appears.

In this scenario, you particularly want to know whether the client has had any changes in bladder or bowel function since the injury (particularly looking for faecal incontinence or urinary retention); whether he is having any anaesthesia or paraesthesia in the saddle area; whether he has noticed any sexual dysfunction; or whether he has any loss of control or sensation in his legs (cauda equina symptoms). You should also be interested in whether he has noticed any unexplained weight loss recently, which may lead you to consider a serious underlying pathology.

Has he had this condition before? If so, how long ago, what was the treatment and what was the outcome?

Past medical history (PMH)

This includes details of any ongoing medical conditions as well as any significant history of medical conditions. You also need to ask about significant surgical history. You might need to spend longer than you imagine on this as some clients may not recall immediately the details of their history, or even their ongoing conditions. You may need to revisit this again once you have the drug history – they don't always match!

Drug history (DH)

This includes not only prescribed medication, but over-the-counter, herbal and recreational medication too. Make sure you are clear about whether the client takes the medication as prescribed/advised.

Note whether the client has any allergies. You could include substances other than drugs, for example food. Also consider whether there could be any interaction between his existing medication and any that you may be about to recommend.

Social history (SH)

Social history is important for you to know about if you are going to advise the client on a management plan. It includes topics such as living accommodation and circumstances.

Who does he live with? What kind of accommodation (house/bungalow/stairs)? Does he work? If so, what does he do (this may affect your advice)? Does he have any hobbies or sporting interests? Does he look after anyone (is he a carer)? If so, what impact is this having on him? Is the condition affecting his ability to carry out his daily activities? Again there will be specific questions you will need to ask depending on the answers given by the client.

You also may want to ask about smoking and alcohol intake. Do not assume that everyone is familiar with the concept of units of alcohol. Instead you may want to ask them how many glasses/pints he drinks in a week and then calculate the units yourself.

Family history (FH)

It may be useful to get an overview of the client's family health here. Are there any medical conditions in the family? Of central importance to include is his birth mother and father; brothers and sisters; and children.

Review of systems (ROS)

This is an opportunity to ask some general questions about the client's health in order to ensure you have not missed anything. This is important because when you and your client talk to each other, it is possible that you both filter out the things you do not feel are relevant to the conversation. This can occasionally lead to important symptoms being missed. You need to cover the major systems (cardiovascular, respiratory, gastrointestinal, genitourinary, neurological and musculoskeletal). A few direct questions about each are adequate, for example, for cardiovascular you could ask whether the client has had any chest pain or palpitations recently; and for respiratory you may ask whether the client has had any shortness of breath or a productive cough.

Once you have completed the history did you recap on the important points to ensure that you understood the client's answers?

You should then have had a discussion with your client about your recommendations. In this case, provided the history was thorough, you could have advised him on analgesics and activity and asked him to review the situation if there was no improvement in a couple of days. It is important to make sure that this is a discussion, not a set of instructions, because the client needs to be in agreement with the proposed action(s) for there to be a satisfactory outcome. In this case, the occupation of the client it likely to be a factor in the management so you need to be prepared to answer questions he may have on this.

Suggested revision points

- Clinical history-taking
- Communication skills
- Management of low back pain
- Cauda equina syndrome.

Scenario 2.2 Respiratory assessment

Format: Interactive station

Supporting material available to student: *BNF*, stethoscope, cleansing hand-gel

Time allowed: 10 minutes

Suggested years of study: Undergraduate years 3–4; preregistration; postgraduate.

Knowledge and skills tested

- Assessment of the respiratory system, demonstrating knowledge and understanding
- Application of clinical examination techniques
- Interpretation of data collected during client examination
- Communication skills.

Task

You are working in a community pharmacy and a 56-year-old woman attends, reporting difficulty in breathing. A primary survey does not reveal any immediate threat to the woman's life and having collected a structured clinical history you believe the client may have a lower respiratory tract infection. From this information you decide that the next step is to carry out a clinical assessment of her respiratory system.

Scenario 2.2 feedback

Before you read the feedback, jot down the processes you would go through and what questions you would ask and why.

How effective was communication during assessment and examination?

Assessment of the respiratory system requires effective client interaction and communication skills by pharmacists. Your communication should be professional, appropriate and effective throughout the station.

Did you obtain consent throughout your client contact?

Remember, consent is a dynamic process, and you are required to obtain consent throughout your client contact. You must gain consent before starting the clinical assessment. You may also need to re-affirm consent during your assessment as some elements may be considered more intrusive than other. Always explain what you are going to do to the client before you do it!

Were key points from the client's history explored?

- Determine the duration of symptoms – is there an acute, acute-on-chronic or chronic illness?
- Can the client describe their symptoms? Are significant features present (e.g. an audible expiratory wheeze)? If

applicable, are these similar or different to prior episodes?

■ Are any associated symptoms such as a cough or pain present? When found, these symptoms require further exploration, considering broader diagnoses – both raise the suspicion of involvement of other system(s) and/or pathologies. Heart failure is a good example of this as it may present predominantly with non-specific and/or respiratory symptoms.

■ Clients unable to provide any history due to respiratory distress (e.g. an adult who cannot complete a sentence without becoming breathless) suggest a serious pathology. Call for ambulance service assistance early.

■ Remember that a structured and comprehensive clinical history (see Scenario 2.1), provided by the client, underpins your assessment and examination of clients.

Examples of respiratory conditions

Specific examples of respiratory conditions relating to asthma and chronic obstructive pulmonary disease (COPD) presentations (two frequently encountered complex respiratory diseases) are explored below.

Asthma Current national guidelines identify the diagnosis of asthma as a clinical process, mandating sophisticated respiratory system assessment and examination skills to be utilised by pharmacists. Unlike other pathophysiological processes, there is an absence of diagnostic tests to identify asthma. Instead asthma is identified by the presence of one or more typical symptoms (wheeze, breathlessness, chest tightness and cough), that when present are accompanied by variable airflow obstruction.

Clinical indications that may support the diagnosis of asthma include:

■ at least one, or more, of typical asthma symptoms (wheeze, cough, difficulty in breathing, chest tightness), particularly if they are:
  – frequent and recurrent
  – worse at night and in the early morning

- provoked by exercise or other triggers (e.g. animals, cold or damp air, emotion or laughter)
- present in the absence of a cold

- known atopic disorder, either personal or familial atopic disease and/or asthma
- presence of a generalised wheeze upon auscultation
- improvement of symptoms or lung function following adequate therapy

Clinical features that do not support diagnosis of asthma include:

- symptoms associated with a 'cold' alone – no symptoms between infections
- cough alone – without wheeze or difficulty breathing
- moist cough
- prominent features of dizziness, light-headedness or peripheral tingling
- normal physical examination of chest when symptomatic
- investigations (peak expiratory flow) or spirometry normal when symptomatic
- appropriate trial therapy for asthma that fails to produce a response.

Chronic obstructive pulmonary disease (COPD)   Like asthma, the suspicion of COPD should be raised from clinical history and presenting clinical features. Consider the diagnosis in people:

- who are aged over 35 years **and**
- smoke or are ex-smokers **and**
- have any of the following symptoms:

  - breathlessness on exertion
  - chronic cough
  - regularly produce sputum
  - frequent episodes of winter 'bronchitis'
  - wheezing

- without features suggesting asthma.

Examination

Examination of the respiratory system is not limited to the chest or lungs – you are required to examine for associated signs to guide your diagnosis. The clinical examination of the respiratory system should include the following aspects:

- *Initial approach to the client*: Rapidly form a decision regarding the appropriateness to continue examination or seek immediate help from a general practitioner and/or call an emergency ambulance. Clients may present with serious respiratory pathologies; candidates can overlook the fact that clients sometimes require urgent transfer to an emergency department. Signs of respiratory distress which would require you to refer the client for assessment in an emergency department include:

  - inability to complete sentences
  - use of the accessory muscles for respiration
  - recession of the thorax between intercostal spaces
  - oxygen saturations measured as less than 95%
  - respiratory rate less than 12 or greater than 20 breaths per minute
  - peripheral and/or central cyanosis
  - reduced level of consciousness
  - significant chest or back trauma.

- *Undertaking a rapid general inspection*: This provides clues as to potential respiratory pathologies and/or alternative disease processes. It should include inspection of:

  - fingers/hands
  - arms/neck
  - eyes
  - mouth.

- *Examination of the thorax*: This comprises four components – inspection, palpation, percussion and auscultation. Candidates sometimes forget that each component of examination must be repeated when examining the anterior, the lateral and the posterior aspects. Consider how you will complete this process while avoiding excessive or repetitive client movement. For example, usually healthcare professionals assess all of the four components of respiratory assessment at each site before moving to another. In the clinical practice environment you will observe practitioners undertaking examination of the respiratory system using various techniques. This is based upon their experience; as a novice, it is important to undertake examinations in the prescribed format.

The four components of the examination of the thorax are described in detail below.

1. Inspection   Do not forget to compare symmetry on both sides of the client's chest. This is to determine abnormalities during respiratory system examination.

During inspection observe carefully for the following signs:

- Assess the work of breathing to determine if clients are utilising increased effort. This can be identified by:

  - accessory muscle utilisation
  - inter/subcostal recession – these are particularly concerning signs; in children they represent impending respiratory failure
  - an abnormal respiratory rate (to avoid influencing the client's rate of breathing, record this while palpating a radial pulse)
  - client's colour – assume signs such as pallor, cyanosis and/or diaphoresis to require assessment by a medical physician.

- Shape of the chest wall, paying particular attention to:

  - whether or not the chest expands and reduces symmetrically
  - presence of surgical scars
  - abnormal chest physiology that can impair thoracic capacity, such as barrel or pigeon shapes.

2. Palpation   Use firm but gentle therapeutic touch to examine for:

- symmetrical chest expansion
- areas of tenderness.

3. Percussion   This is a difficult skill to master, requiring practice relating to technique of eliciting the sign and interpreting the results. You should percuss the same number of sites as for auscultation (e.g. six anterior, six posterior and a triangle of three sites on the lateral aspect of the client). Possible findings include:

- normal resonance
- hyper-resonance which may signify pneumothorax
- dullness which may signify pulmonary effusion or consolidation.

4. Auscultation   Regular practice with a stethoscope is essential to accurately identify these sounds. Consider the underpinning anatomy and use a variety of sites – as you do in percussion. You should determine the presence or absence of:

- vesicular breath sounds
- wheezing
- stridor
- crepitation – differentiating between fine and coarse.

Before forming a management plan

Have you considered the need for further or supplemental diagnostic tests? These may include:

- near client testing such as end-tidal carbon dioxide measurement, peak expiratory flow
- further tests such as spirometry or an electrocardiogram (ECG).

These may need to be arranged via a client's GP or other clinician competent in the interpretation of the results.

Suggested revision points

- Assessment techniques including communication skills and a broad repertoire of investigative questions
- Terminology relevant to the assessment of clients
- The examination skills of respiratory examination:
  - inspection
  - palpation of the anterior, lateral and posterior chest
  - percussion using a variety of sites
  - auscultation using the same sites as percussion
- Knowledge of respiratory system pathologies and examination findings.

Scenario 2.3 Cardiac emergency

Format: Interactive station

Supporting material available to student: *BNF*, stethoscope, cleansing hand-gel

Time allowed: 5 minutes

Suggested years of study: Undergraduate years 2–4; preregistration; postgraduate.

Knowledge and skills tested

- Use of a global overview and focused history-taking in patient assessment
- Knowledge of cardiac emergencies
- Taking emergency action
- Communication skills.

Task

While you are working in a community pharmacy, a 66-year-old man, who is overweight, comes in for a consultation regarding persistent indigestion. The man looks extremely pale in colour and is sweating profusely. You are required to take a clinical history from this client, and make recommendations as appropriate.

Scenario 2.3 feedback

You should introduce yourself and gain consent to take a clinical history from this client. When you ask him about his presenting complaint he tells you:

- He woke up that morning with indigestion-like pain in his upper abdomen.
- The pain has persisted despite taking over-the-counter antacids.
- The pain has increased.
- He has a feeling of pressure in his chest.

Although you are taking an oral history, you still need to use observation skills to note your client's condition. It is clear that he is extremely pale in colour and that he is sweating profusely. This client's presentation suggests acute coronary syndrome (ACS) and this client may be having a myocardial infarction.

Your assessment of the client should STOP at this point and you should take the following actions:

- Calmly communicate your concerns to the client.
- Acquire their consent to dial 999 for an ambulance, ensuring that you inform the ambulance service call-taker that the client has chest pain and that you suspect he is having a heart attack.
- Keep the client comfortable and reassured by communicating appropriately with him. It is advisable not to leave him on his own.
- If possible find someone who is competent at Basic Life Support in case the client collapses. If there is an automated external defibrillator (AED) available, this should be accessed promptly if the client collapses.

Key points for a focused assessment in a time critical emergency:

- It is vital to establish exactly what the client's presenting complaint is, and fully explore any associated symptoms early on in any client encounter so as to quickly identify those clients who have potentially life-threatening conditions.
- You must be aware of 'red flags' that may become apparent during either your history-taking or clinical examination of any client and how to respond appropriately.
- Remember the importance of gaining a global overview of the client early on in the encounter. This means balancing what you are being told by the client with what you can observe about the client. In the above scenario the client appears pale and sweaty and complains of indigestion-like pain and tightness in the chest. This in itself is enough to strongly suggest a heart attack. Balanced with the client's age and weight this makes him particularly high risk for acute coronary syndrome.
- Taking the client's complaint of 'indigestion' at face value and not being thorough in establishing exactly what the client is experiencing and balancing this with the client's overall appearance would be a major error in this situation.
- Continuing with any further assessment of this client prior to taking the appropriate emergency action (999) would be potentially fatal for this client.

Suggested revision points

- Signs and symptoms of ACS
- How to make a 999 call
- Basic Life Support
- The role of AED in the management of cardiac arrest
- Role of aspirin in cardiac events.

Scenario 2.4 Focused history-taking and neurological assessment

Format: Interactive station

Supporting material available to student: *BNF*, blood pressure monitor, tympanic thermometer, stethoscope, cleansing hand-gel

Time allowed: 20 minutes

Suggested years of study: Undergraduate years 3–4; pre-registration; postgraduate.

Knowledge and skills tested

- Use of global overview followed by focused client history
- Knowledge of primary and secondary causes of headaches
- Recognition of 'red flags'
- Selection of appropriate clinical examinations
- Communication skills.

Task

While you are working in a community pharmacy, a 48-year-old man presents to you wanting advice on analgesia because he is experiencing episodic, daily, tight 'band-like' headaches. He is orientated, looks well with no apparent neurological deficit. He has recently been promoted at work. You are required to take a history and undertake any other assessments you consider necessary.

Scenario 2.4 feedback

Before you read the feedback, jot down the processes you would go through and what questions you would ask and why.

Did you use your observations skills here? The fact that this client has presented to you (not his GP), that he is orientated, and he looks well, are less worrying signs. Successful management of headaches relies on gathering a good systematic history, taking time to elicit the pertinent features of the headache. Headaches affect a large proportion of the UK population at least occasionally. The vast majority are benign and self-limiting. Do not be overconfident, work within your diagnostic scope of practice, and if in doubt refer.

You need to establish whether this is a primary or secondary cause headache. Table 2.1 gives some examples of each. Primary cause headaches can be elicited on the basis of a good history; there are no confirmatory tests or procedures. Secondary cause headaches are more worrying, often heralding serious underlying pathology; they usually require onward referral.

So the first action is to undertake a systematic clinical history. In this example, we will use a focused clinical history as opposed to covering all elements as we did in Scenario 2.1:

- Did you introduce yourself and gain consent before you started the history-taking and any physical examinations?
- Start by asking open-ended questions. Does the client usually experience headaches? If so why are they consulting now? IMPORTANT: use a separate history for each type of headache that the client experiences.

Table 2.1 Examples of primary and secondary cause headaches

Primary cause	Secondary cause
Tension-type headache (TTH)	Subarachnoid haemorrhage (SAH)
Migraine	Trauma
Cluster	Space-occupying lesion (SOL)
	Meningitis
	From eyes, teeth and neck
	Temporal arteritis (giant cell arteritis – GCA)

Presenting complaint and history of presenting complaint (PC and HPC)

Sometimes these two areas overlap and the client may move from one to the other during dynamic communication, but you need to make sure you have covered all of these areas during the history-taking.

- Where is the headache? Tension headaches tend to be diffuse 'like a tight band' or 'skullcap'. Migraines are more likely unilateral and pulsating. Cluster headaches tend to be located over one eye and are more common in males aged above 20 years, often occurring at night for a period of weeks then subsiding for several months. Pain over the temples with accompanying scalp tenderness in clients aged over 50 years is indicative of temporal arteritis – refer urgently for appropriate treatment.
- When did it start? A sudden onset of 'worst headache ever' is of great concern, particularly in the occipital region and it is often described as 'like being hit with a bat'. Treat this as a subarachnoid haemorrhage (SAH), dial 999 and call for paramedic assistance.
- Has the client suffered any trauma? Consider post-concussion syndrome or potential intracranial haemorrhage.
- Does the pain occur at the same time of day, perhaps after work? Potentially a tension-type headache (TTH).
- Has the person had it before? Recurrent headaches tend to be less sinister, as are headaches occurring in predictable patterns. Be suspicious of the client complaining of persistent headache exacerbated by lying down, especially if accompanied by early morning nausea. This should be considered a space-occupying lesion (SOL) and referred urgently. Migraines can become recognisable to those who experience them. Classic migraine presents with an aura lasting between 5 and 60 minutes, such as a jagged crescent (scintillating scotoma); nausea, vomiting, photophobia, phonophobia (aversion to noise) can also be present.

- What is the character of the pain? Does anything provoke or palliate it? Does the pain change with coughing, straining or sneezing? If so, again suspect an SOL and refer urgently. Ask about neck pain during movements, enquire about tenderness and stiffness – possible cervico-genic headache. Does the pain respond to analgesia? If not, reconsider a less serious diagnosis. Persistent, progressive, unremitting pain is almost always a marker of serious underlying pathology requiring investigation.

Past medical history and drug history (PMH and DH)

Certain drugs such as glyceryl trinitrate and calcium channel blockers can cause headaches. Medication overuse headache (MOH) is more common in women and is highly variable, oppressive and often presents on waking. Females who experience migraine especially with aura are at increased risk of stroke when taking the combined oral contraceptive pill (COCP), so remember to enquire about this during the drug history.

Any systemic features present?

Undertake a brief review of systems (ROS). Ask the client about fever, malaise, myalgia, or night sweats suggestive of an infectious pathology such as meningitis. Enquire about any weight loss indicating possible malignancy. Ask about nausea and vomiting, 'fits, faints and funny turns' and visual problems.

Key features of headaches are described in Box 2.1.

Box 2.1   Summary of headaches

Primary cause headache

- *Tension-type headaches (TTH)*: Episodic with variable pattern. Lasts several hours (but no more). Pressing 'band-like'/'skull cap' diffuse pain. Non-disabling. Responds well to simple analgesia. Can develop into chronic type >15 days per month.

- *Migraine*: Episodic and lasts a few hours up to 3 days. Unilateral pain described as pulsating. Affects 15% of the population, women more commonly. Can cause visual disturbances between 5 and 60 minutes before onset of headache. Clients are often aware of known triggers. Activity is severely restricted during attacks; clients often seek a quiet, dark room until symptoms pass. Can also present with nausea, vomiting, photophobia and phonophobia. Migraine has several overlap symptoms with more serious secondary headaches such as rapid onset, vomiting, photophobia and 'worse headache ever'. This may explain why migraine is the most common primary headache disorder seen in the emergency department. If in doubt – refer.

- *Cluster headache*: Intermittent severe pain located over/around one eye occurring in 'clusters' of around 30–60 minutes with remissions. Often at night; affects young males more commonly. Clients often present with agitation and pacing.

Secondary cause headache

- *Subarachnoid haemorrhage (SAH)*: Sudden onset, explosive occipital headache with photophobia, nausea and neck stiffness.

- *Temporal arteritis*: Generally older than 50 years with scalp tenderness ± pain over temples. Other features include malaise, jaw/muscle pain and visual disturbance.

- *Space-occupying lesion (SOL)*: Dull headache, worse in the morning ± nausea. Subtle personality changes or problems with memory and reasoning. Headache that changes with position, coughing and straining.

- *Traumatic cause*: Pain lessens from time of incident but can cause anxiety and increased psycho-social morbidity. Intracranial bleeding should be suspected if presenting with nausea, vomiting, seizures and focal neurology.

Red flags (symptoms which should not be ignored and need urgent medical advice)

- Thunderclap: sudden explosive onset
- Atypical aura (>1 hour ± motor weakness)
- Aura for first time during oral contraceptive use

- New onset <10 years >50 years
- Progressive, worsening over weeks or longer
- Associated with postural change
- New onset with previous medical history of carcinoma or HIV
- New or unexpected in an individual client
- Neck stiffness
- Loss of consciousness (LOC) (however transient)
- Fit/collapse
- Visual disturbance
- Focal neurological deficit
- Changes in memory, personality or reasoning
- Worse on waking
- 'First and worst'.

Having taken a clinical history, consider whether a clinical examination is required.

- *Blood pressure*: Consider the client's fears. They may be concerned about serious pathologies and blood pressure is rarely a cause (unless secondary hypertension), but clients may expect to have their blood pressure measured.
- *Temperature*: This can be taken quickly and easily using a tympanic thermometer. If raised, consider a different or more serious pathology.
- *Cranial nerve examination*: This is essential. Pay particular attention to the eyes (H-test) and pupillary reaction. Observe for ptosis (drooping eyelid), exophthalmos (bulging of the eye anteriorly out of the orbit), miosis (constricted pupil). A cloudy cornea with or without visual halos is indicative of glaucoma. Mydriasis (dilated pupil) can indicate a subarachnoid haemorrhage (SAH).
- *Fundoscopy*: This requires the use of an ophthalmoscope, which requires considerable skill to perform correctly.

Look for papilloedema – a sign of raised intracranial pressure.

- *Horner's syndrome*: This deserves a special mention. It occurs as a result of an ipsilateral (same side) sympathetic nerve problem. It presents with a triad of ptosis, miosis and anhydrosis (dry skin around the orbit). Make sure you enquire about neck pain (carotid artery dissection) but refer this client to a doctor regardless of whether or not they have neck pain.
- Check for photophobia (dislike of bright light), neck stiffness, limb strength and coordination. You will have established during the history whether the client is orientated and responding appropriately.

Suggested revision points

- Core elements of systematic clinical history-taking
- Appropriate selection of areas for a focused clinical history
- Knowledge of primary and secondary causes of headaches
- Knowledge of a variety of neurological clinical examinations
- Recognition and understanding of relevant neurological 'red flags'
- Communication skills.

Scenario 2.5 Monitoring blood glucose

Format: Interactive station

Supporting material available to student: Glucometer and test strips, lancets and administrator, alcohol wipes, cotton wool, sharps box, gloves, cleansing hand-gel

Time allowed: 5 minutes

Suggested years of study: Undergraduate years 2–4; pre-registration; postgraduate.

Knowledge and skills tested

- Safe management of blood glucometer including calibration
- Awareness of normal blood glucose range
- Awareness of management and/or advice for people who are hypoglycaemic or hyperglycaemic
- Safe handling of blood products and disposal of sharps
- Accurate and appropriate recording of relevant data
- Communication skills.

Task

A 55-year-old woman has asked to have her blood glucose levels assessed. You are required to perform this procedure.

Scenario 2.5 feedback

Before you read the feedback, jot down here how you would approach this situation.

Prior to carrying out this procedure, all necessary equipment should be checked, this should also involve the calibration of your particular blood glucose monitor with the corresponding blood test strips. This procedure must be carried out prior to the test being undertaken as both measuring tool and strip must be compatible. (Please refer to manufacturers' instructions.)

Glucose monitoring is an invasive technique that requires the client's consent prior to the procedure being undertaken.

Did you follow the procedure below?

- Even if the client is used to this procedure, you should still explain it to them.
- Turn on the glucose monitor and ensure it is calibrated.
- Clean the client's finger with an alcohol wipe and allow it to dry.

- Prepare the test strip, making sure it is in date and in good condition.
- Prick the client's finger with the lancet and dispose of the lancet into the sharps bin.
- Squeeze the finger gently and then position the finger over the test strip so that the blood drops on to the test strip.
- Give the client a cotton wool ball and press firmly on the pricked site to stop any further bleeding.
- Note the reading from the glucometer.
- Inform the client of the reading.
- Document the reading and take appropriate action according to the result.

Suggested revision points

- Familiarisation with blood glucometers, including calibration
- Awareness of suitable sites to target for collection of capillary blood
- Awareness of safe disposal of sharps
- Understanding of 'normal' range of blood glucose
- Knowledge of what constitutes hypoglycaemia and hyperglycaemia and what advice needs to be given to clients presenting with either of these
- Knowledge of action to be taken in a hypoglycaemic emergency
- Communication skills.

Scenario 2.6 Monitoring a radial pulse

Format: Interactive station

Supporting material available to student: cleansing hand-gel, a watch that gives time in seconds

Time allowed: 5 minutes

Suggested years of study: Undergraduate years 1–4; pre-registration; postgraduate.

Knowledge and skills tested

- Accurate location of a radial arterial pulse
- Accurate measurement of a pulse rate using the appropriate pulse point
- Recognition of the strength and regularity of the pulse
- Appropriate length of time given to make a record
- Accurate and appropriate recording of relevant data
- Communication skills.

Task

An 18-year-old woman presents to you stating that she has had a sudden sense of anxiety and feels that her pulse 'is racing'. She has no significant medical history and the onset of symptoms appears to be acute and without obvious cause. The client appears fit and well. Please take a radial pulse measurement and record that measurement.

Scenario 2.6 feedback

Before you read the feedback, jot down here how you would undertake this.

Having suggested that you wish to take their pulse, the client should be reassured and their consent obtained for the examination.

- The client should be seated and given time to relax.
- The client's arm should be positioned so that she is comfortable – palm upwards.
- The radial pulse is anatomically convenient for measurement and is, generally, the easiest to palpate.
- The radial pulse should be the pulse point of choice under these circumstances.
- The radial pulse should be palpated using your first and second digits without excessive pressure that might occlude the artery.

- The length of time taken to measure the rate needs to be appropriate to the client condition (e.g. if slow rate a full minute should be taken to get a recording).
- The rate and qualitative data (strength and regularity) need to be accurately documented.
- Always inform the client of the results, as it can be worrying to clients if that information is withheld.

Suggested revision points

- Familiarisation with the anatomy of the wrist
- Knowledge of alternative pulse point locations
- Knowledge of normal pulse rates
- Knowledge of normal and irregular pulse rhythm and strength
- Practise palpating pulse points and calculating pulse rates.

Scenario 2.7 Measuring respiration rate

Format: Interactive station

Supporting material available to student: A watch that shows the time in seconds

Time allowed: 5 minutes

Suggested years of study: Undergraduate years 1–4; pre-registration; postgraduate.

Knowledge and skills tested

- Accurate measurement of a client's respiratory rate
- Recognition of any abnormal rate and/or breath sounds
- Appropriate length of time taken to observe respiration
- Accurate and appropriate recording of relevant data
- Communication skills.

Task

You are asked to assess the respiration rate of a client who has presented in your pharmacy complaining of slight shortness of breath.

Scenario 2.7 feedback

Before you read the feedback, jot down here what you would do in this situation.

- The client should be reassured and consent sought for the examination.
- The client should be seated and given time to relax.
- Respiratory rate can be easily influenced by the client due to the practitioner's observation, so this is best monitored surreptitiously while appearing to take a radial pulse rate.
- Observe abdominal movement if chest rise is not obvious.
- If there is a slow respiration rate, take a full minute to make the recording.
- Note the character of the breath sounds as well as the rate.
- Note any abnormal physical effort required for breathing, such as use of accessory muscles.
- The respiration rate and any qualitative data (for example regularity, depth) need to be accurately documented.

Suggested revision points

- Knowledge of normal breathing rates at rest
- Knowledge of abnormal breath sounds
- Knowledge of associated abnormal physical effort when breathing
- Practise observing and calculating respiration rates.

Scenario 2.8 Using a binaural acoustic stethoscope

Format: Interactive station

Supporting material available to student: Binaural acoustic stethoscope, alcohol wipes

Time allowed: 5 minutes

Suggested years of study: Undergraduate years 1–4; pre-registration; postgraduate.

Knowledge and skills tested

- Appropriate use of a binaural acoustic stethoscope
- Safe use of a binaural acoustic stethoscope
- Communication skills.

Task

You are going to use the binaural acoustic stethoscope as part of your client's assessment.

Scenario 2.8 feedback

Before you read the feedback, consider how you would proceed in this situation.

- The ear pieces should be cleaned, as needed, using alcohol solution.
- The bell is rotated with the diaphragm down (i.e. for client contact).

- Consent should be gained before proceeding with the examination.
- The procedure is explained to the client to maximise compliance.
- Strategies for overcoming communication difficulties during the auscultation should be explained to your client before you start. For example, if they want to get your attention they should touch your arm or shoulder.
- The ear pieces should be correctly orientated (i.e. the ear tubes should point angled in a forward direction as you insert them into your ear canals).
- Extraneous sounds are avoided (for example, anything rubbing against tubing) and the procedure is conducted in a quiet environment.
- Warm the bell and diaphragm before skin contact if in a cool/cold environment.
- The stethoscope should be appropriately placed on the client for whichever assessment is being undertaken.

Suggested revision points

- Familiarise yourself with the stethoscope's individual parts
- Practise using the stethoscope
- Refer to particular assessment procedures where the use of the stethoscope is required so that correct for placement of the stethoscope bell is made.

Chapter 2 feedback summary

In Chapter 2 we have explored a variety of activities related to client assessment. Please remember that what is being offered here is merely an introduction to some of the core elements of clinical history-taking and client assessment. You should refer to the reference list provided for further reading to help guide

Table 2.2 Chapter 2 learning outcomes

Knowledge and skills	More work required	Feel competent
Systematic clinical history-taking		
Respiratory assessment		
Recognising an emergency cardiac event		
Neurological assessment		
Use of a stethoscope		
Blood glucose measurement		
Monitoring a pulse		
Monitoring respiration rate		
Formulate a working diagnosis		
Offer appropriate advice to clients		

you to further learning and development in this expansive area of professional practice.

Now that you have completed this chapter, assess your competence in the knowledge and skills listed in Table 2.2. Jot down any notes that may help you.

If there are any points that you consider need further work, start a CPD (continuous professional development) cycle now to identify how you can achieve this action.

References and further reading

Bowker LK, Price JD, Smith SC (2006). *The Essential Hands on Guide to the Care of Older Clients. Oxford Handbook of Geriatric Medicine.* Oxford: Oxford University Press.

British Thoracic Society/Scottish Intercollegiate Guidelines Network (2011). *British Guidelines on the Management of Asthma: a national clinical guideline*, revised edn. Available from http://www.brit-thoracic.org.uk/Portals/0/Guidelines/AsthmaGuidelines/sign101%20Sept%202011.pdf (accessed 6 June 2012).

Carroll L (2007). *Acute Medicine: A handbook for nurse practitioners.* Chichester: Wiley.

Cox N, Roper TA (2005). *Clinical Skills.* Oxford: Oxford University Press.

Devereux G, Douglas G (2008). Examination of the respiratory system. In Douglas G, Nicol F, Robertson C, eds. *Macleod's Clinical Examination*, 11th edn. Elsevier: Edinburgh, pp. 123–152.

Farne H, Norris-Cervetto E, Warbrick-Smith, J (2010). *Oxford Cases in Medicine and Surgery.* Oxford: Oxford University Press.

Hopcroft K, Forte V (2010). *Symptom Sorter*, 4th edn. Abingdon: Radcliffe Pubishing.

McMurray J, Petrie M, Swedberg K, Komajda M, Anker S, Gardner R (2009). Heart failure. In Camm AJ, Luscher TF, Serruys PW, eds. *The ESC Textbook of Cardiovascular Medicine*, 2nd edn. Oxford: Oxford University Press, chapter 23.

NHS National Institute for Health and Clinical Excellence (2010). *CG101 Chronic Obstructive Pulmonary Disease (update): quick reference guide.* Available from http://www.nice.org.uk/nicemedia/live/13029/49399/49399.pdf (accessed 6 June 2012).

Richards D, Aronso J (2005) *How to Prescribe Safely and Effectively. Oxford Handbook of Practical Drug Therapy.* Oxford: Oxford University Press.

Souhami RL, Moxham J (2002). *Textbook of Medicine*, 4th edn. Edinburgh: Churchill Livingstone.

Woollard M, Greaves I (2008). Shortness of breath. In Wardrope J, Driscoll P, Laird C, Woollard M, eds. *Community Emergency Medicine: A system of assessment and care pathways.* Oxford: Elsevier, pp. 53–74.

3

Legal aspects of prescriptions, and record-keeping

Beti Wyn Evans and Nina Walker

Chapter 3 includes scenarios that assess knowledge and application of legal aspects of prescriptions and of dispensing. This includes controlled drugs and private prescriptions.

Before you embark on the following scenarios, ensure that you know prescription requirements, record-keeping requirements for prescription-only medicines (POMs) including controlled drugs (CDs), and emergency supply of POMs.

Key references

Joint Formulary Committee. *British National Formulary*. London: BMJ Group and Pharmaceutical Press (introductory chapters).
Royal Pharmaceutical Society (2012). *Medicines, Ethics and Practice*. Available to members from the Royal Pharmaceutical Society from www.rpharms.com (accessed 28 May 2012).

Learning objectives

The following OSCE scenarios assess record-keeping skills. By the end of this chapter you should be able to:

- record supply of a POM ordered on a private prescription
- record a supply of CDs
- record emergency supply of a POM at the request of a patient
- record emergency supply of a POM at the request of a prescriber.

Scenario 3.1 Private prescription

Format: Written station

Supporting material available to student: Medicines, Ethics and Practice guide, *BNF*

Time allowed: 5 minutes

Suggested years of study: Undergraduate years 1–4; pre-registration.

Knowledge and skills tested

- Knowledge of legal prescription requirements
- Record-keeping requirements for private prescriptions.

Task

A patient brings a private prescription to you in the pharmacy. The details on the prescription are listed below. You are required to make an appropriate pharmacy record for this prescription, including all necessary legal and professional requirements. You make the supply of the medication today.

The following details are written on the prescription:

Dr FD Jenkins MBBS, MRCP
The Surgery
Anytown AN9 6NE
Rx

Mr Edward Bennett
1 High Street
Anytown AN9 3GB

3rd June 2012

Propranolol tablets 40 mg b.d.
Mitte 56

J D Jenkins

Scenario 3.1 feedback

You should have learned the legal and professional requirements for private prescriptions within pharmacy practice dispensing classes. In this scenario you are expected to interpret the prescription provided and then make an appropriate record on a blank sheet of paper from a POM register. Remember to check the validity of the prescription.

In the practice situation, before you dispense a private prescription, you may wish to confirm the prescriber's General Medical Council registration, especially if the prescriber is not known to you. Prescribers should be 'registered with a licence to practise'.

The necessary information to be recorded for the prescription is provided below:

- *Date of supply*: Add today's date (the date of the assessment), unless you are told otherwise in the scenario or brief.
- *Prescription date*: 3rd June 2012 (that is, the date the prescription was written).
- *Patient details*: Mr Edward Bennett, 1 High Street, Anytown AN9 3GB.
- *Prescriber details*: Dr FD Jenkins MBBS, MRCP, The Surgery, Anytown AN9 6NE.
- *Medication details*: Propranolol tablets 40 mg b.d. 56 tablets supplied.

It is also good practice to enter a reference number of the prescription in the register. Some pharmacies use a book and page number system. The cost is often recorded too, although this is not a legal requirement for a private prescription register entry.

Suggested revision points

- If you are not sure of the record-keeping requirements, have a look now in the *MEP* (*Medicines Ethics and Practice*) guide. Use this as a checklist for what you should record if you have access to the guide in the OSCE situation.

Practise remembering what legal requirements apply to private prescription entries.
■ Location of prescription records in the workplace.

Scenario 3.2 Controlled drug supply

Format: Written station

Supporting material available to student: *Medicines, Ethics and Practice* guide, *BNF*

Time allowed: 5 minutes

Suggested years of study: Undergraduate years 1–4; pre-registration.

Knowledge and skills tested

■ Knowledge of current CD regulations
■ Ability to record CD supply.

Task

A customer enters your pharmacy on a Sunday afternoon, when the local GP surgeries are closed, and presents an FP10 prescription for oxycodone 5 mg capsules. The prescriber is known to you, the patient receives this medication on a regular basis, and you have no reason to doubt the authenticity of the prescription. List the checks you would make, including any amendments you deem to be necessary, and make an appropriate record (if necessary) in the CD register (Table 3.1).

The details on the prescription are:

Title, Forename, Surname & Address: Mr Andrew North, 1 Main Road, Anytown AN1 2BC
Medication details: Oxycodone 5 mg capsules. Sig 1 b.d. Mitte thirty caps.
Prescriber's details: Dr A Smith, The Surgery, Anytown AN9 2GR

The prescription is signed and is in date.

Table 3.1 CD register

Drug class:		Name/Brand:		Strength:		Form:		Balance
Date supply received or date supplied	Received				Supplied			
	Name and address from whom received	Quantity received	Name and address of person or firm supplied	Detail of authority to possess – prescriber or licence holder's details	Person collecting Schedule 2 controlled drug (patient/ patient's rep/healthcare professional) and, if healthcare professional, name and address	Was proof of identity requested of patient/ patient's rep? (Yes / No)	Was proof of identity of person collecting provided? (Yes / No)	Quantity supplied

Table reproduced with permission from the National Pharmacy Association (NPA); published by NPA, 2008.

Scenario 3.2 feedback

List the checks you would make, including any amendments you deem to be necessary.

The checks you need to make to ensure the prescription requirements are met are:

- name and address of the patient
- name and address of the prescriber
- date (within 28 days)
- name of drug
- quantity (in both words and figures)
- dose
- in the case of a preparation, the form and, where appropriate, strength of the preparation.

Having completed these checks you would have discovered that the total quantity of oxycodone on the prescription is written in words only. The pharmacist is able to amend minor technical errors on Schedule 2 and 3 CD prescriptions. The student should, therefore, add the quantity in figures (in ink), initial the amendment (again, in ink), and make an entry in the CD register.

An example of a completed CD register entry for this prescription is given in Table 3.2. Note that when completing an entry of the supply of a controlled drug, you should leave the 'received' columns blank.

Where do you find out whether records are necessary? The *MEP* guide will tell you the classification of the drug, and the record-keeping requirements thereof.

Suggested revision points

- Record-keeping requirements for CDs
- Amendments that pharmacists are permitted to make to CD prescriptions.

Table 3.2 Completed entry for Scenario 3.2

Drug class: *Oxycodone*	Name/Brand: *Oxynorm®*							Strength: *5mg*	Form: *capsules*
	Received			Supplied					
Date supply received or date supplied	Received	Name and address from whom received	Quantity received	Name and address of person or firm supplied	Detail of authority to possess – prescriber or licence holder's details	Person collecting Schedule 2 controlled drug (patient/ patient's rep/healthcare professional) and, if healthcare professional, name and address	Was proof of identity requested of patient/ patient's rep? (Yes / No)	Was proof of identity of person collecting provided? (Yes / No)	Quantity supplied	Balance
Insert date of assessment				*Mr Andrew North, 1 Main Road, Anytown AN1 2BC*	*Dr A Smith, The Surgery, Anytown AN9 2QR* (NHS prescription)	*Patient* (unless told otherwise in the assessment)	*Yes*	*Yes*	*30*	(leave blank in an OSCE assessment unless you are provided with a partly completed register in which a running total is used)

Scenario 3.3 Managing errors in CD register entries

Format: Written station

Supporting material available to student: *Medicines, Ethics and Practice* guide, *BNF*

Time allowed: 5 minutes

Suggested years of study: Undergraduate years 2–4; pre-registration.

Knowledge and skills tested

- CD record-keeping requirements
- Ability to correct an error in a register entry for CD supply.

Task

You are working in a community pharmacy and dispense the prescription for Zomorph® capsules shown. As required in the CD regulations, you also make an entry into the CD register. Upon checking this, however, you realise you have made a mistake (Table 3.3). You are required to:

1. identify the error
2. correct the error in the entry appropriately.

You should assume that this has all happened today.

> The details on the NHS FP10 prescription are:
>
> Title, forename, surname and address: Mrs Sally Beacon, 9 The Grove, Anytown AN1 7DS
> Medication details: Zomorph® 10 mg capsules. One capsule b.d. Mitte 56 (fifty-six) capsules.
> Prescriber's details: Dr A Smith, The Surgery, Anytown AN9 2GR

Table 3.3 CD register entry for Scenario 3.3

Drug class: *Morphine salts*		Name/Brand: *Zomorph®*		Strength: *10 mg*			Form: *capsules*	
Date supply received or date supplied	*Received*		*Supplied*					*Balance*
	Name and address from whom received	Quantity received	Name and address of person or firm supplied	Detail of authority to possess – prescriber or licence holder's details	Person collecting Schedule 2 controlled drug (patient/ patient's rep/healthcare professional) and, if healthcare professional, name and address	Was proof of identity requested of patient/ patient's rep? (Yes / No)	Was proof of identity of person collecting provided? (Yes / No)	Quantity supplied
Date of assessment			*Mrs Sally Bevan, 9 The Grove, Anytown AN1 7DJ*	*Dr A Smith, The Surgery, Anytown AN9 2SR* (NHS prescription)	*Patient* (unless told otherwise in the assessment)	*Yes*	*Yes*	*56*

Scenario 3.3 feedback

1. Identify the error

Try to be systematic in how you check a CD register entry, working from one side of the register to the other, checking the entry against the prescription details as you go. Do not forget to check the information at the top of the table (i.e. drug class and other details). In this case, the error in the entry is the patient's surname. The surname has been entered as Bevan, when it should read Beacon.

2. Correct the error in the entry appropriately

Do you know how to make amendments in the CD register? If not then find out now. Corrections must be made by footnotes or dated marginal notes. Entries must not be cancelled (crossed-out), obliterated or altered.

It is advised to use an asterix or key to identify the mistake, and to write what should have been entered in the footnote or margin. It is good practice to initial or sign, and date the correction.

Note that when completing an entry of the supply of a controlled drug, you should leave the 'received' columns blank.

Suggested revision points

■ Practise making and correcting CD register entries.

Scenario 3.4 Emergency supply at the request of a prescriber

Format: Interactive station

Supporting material available to student: *Medicines, Ethics and Practice* guide, *BNF*

Time allowed: 5 minutes

Suggested years of study: Undergraduate years 1–4; pre-registration.

Knowledge and skills tested

- The legal conditions applicable to undertaking an emergency supply at the request of a prescriber
- Record-keeping requirements for an emergency supply at the request of a prescriber
- Telephone communication skills.

Task

You have just finished a consultation with a patient in your pharmacy when your colleague passes you a message to telephone Dr A Smith. Dr Smith is a local GP you know well. He is visiting a patient at her home, and wishes to request an emergency supply of a POM.

- What information should you obtain from Dr Smith?
- Decide whether it is appropriate to make the supply and, if so, obtain the necessary details in order to make a valid entry in the prescription-only medicine register.

The doctor provides the following information:

- The doctor's name is Dr Alan Smith, The Surgery, High Street, Anytown AN1 2TF (he is also the prescriber).
- He wishes to request an emergency supply for a patient.
- Patient's name: Elizabeth Green
- Patient's address: 1 Olympic Drive, Anytown AN1 5QW
- Patient's age: 71 years
- Particulars of medicine: Trimethoprim 200 mg b.d. for 3 days
- Nature of emergency: Elderly patient lives several miles from surgery. She has been unwell for 24 hours, very high temperature, and it is impractical for her to collect her prescription, or for the GP to deliver the prescription to the pharmacy today.

The doctor says he will furnish a prescription, by hand, tomorrow afternoon on his way through town. The date on the prescription is today's date.

Scenario 3.4 feedback

In order to make an emergency supply at the request of the prescriber, you must:

- be satisfied that the request is from a prescriber who is permitted to make such requests
- be satisfied that there is an emergency and a prescription cannot be provided immediately, however a written prescription will be provided within 72 hours
- supply the medicine in accordance with the direction given by the prescriber.

An entry must be made into the POM register on the day of the supply (or, if impractical, on the next day following).

Did you make an entry in the POM register? You should have done. The information recorded should include the:

- date the POM was supplied
- name (including strength and form where appropriate) and quantity of medicine supplied
- name and address of the prescriber requesting the emergency supply
- name and address of the patient for whom the POM was required
- date on the prescription (this can be added to the entry when the prescription is received by the pharmacy)
- date on which the prescription is received (this should be added to the entry when the prescription is received in the pharmacy)
- a reference number (good practice).

Therefore to be able to record this information, you need to ask for this in any telephone consultation with the prescriber.

Remember that stations involving the use of the telephone may assess your communication skills. If you are telephoning the prescriber, make sure you confirm who you are speaking to when you initiate the conversation. Do not forget to introduce yourself, and to remind the prescriber why you are calling. It is useful to confirm all details at the end of the consultation so you can correct any errors and/or remind yourself of information you have forgotten to ask for.

Suggested revision points

■ Emergency supply at the request of the prescriber.

Scenario 3.5 Emergency supply at the request of a patient

Format: Written station

Supporting material available to student: *Medicines, Ethics and Practice* guide, *BNF*

Time allowed: 5 minutes

Suggested years of study: Undergraduate years 1–4; preregistration.

Knowledge and skills tested

■ The legal conditions applicable to undertaking an emergency supply of a POM at the request of a patient
■ Record-keeping requirements for emergency supply at the request of a patient.

Task

A customer enters the pharmacy where you are working late on a Saturday evening and approaches the medicines counter. They state that they have run out completely of their levothyroxine tablets, which they must take every day. The following Monday is a bank holiday, and doctors' surgeries are now closed until Tuesday morning.

You interview the patient, and are satisfied that the requirements for emergency supply at the request of the patient have been met. You make a supply of the required medication.

You are required to record the supply in the POM register. You should assume this has all happened today.

Scenario 3.5 feedback

Your entry in the register should include the following:

- date on which the supply was made
- the name, quantity, and pharmaceutical form and strength (where appropriate), of the medicine
- the patient's name and address
- the nature of the emergency, to include why the patient requires the POM and why a prescription cannot be obtained
- a reference number (good practice).

Note that for quantity of supply, in this case, up to 30 days can be supplied. It is up to you to use professional judgement to supply a reasonable quantity that is clinically appropriate and lasts until the patient is able to see a prescriber to obtain a further supply.

Suggested revision points

- Conditions for emergency supply at the request of a patient
- Record-keeping requirements for emergency supply at the request of a patient.

Chapter 3 feedback summary

In Chapter 3 you have looked at some aspects of legal prescription requirements, and of record-keeping requirements relating to private prescriptions, controlled drugs and emergency supply.

Table 3.4 Chapter 3 learning outcomes

Knowledge and skills	More work required	Feel competent
Record supply of a POM ordered on a private prescription		
Record a supply of controlled drugs		
Record emergency supply of a POM at the request of a prescriber		
Record emergency supply of a POM at the request of a patient		

Now that you have completed this chapter, assess your competence in the knowledge and skills listed in Table 3.4. Jot down any notes that may help you.

If there are any points that you consider need further work, start a CPD (continuous professional development) cycle now to identify how you can achieve this action.

References and further reading

Royal Pharmaceutical Society of Great Britain (2012). *Medicines, Ethics and Practice*. Edition 36. London: Royal Pharmaceutical Society of Great Britain.

4

Data retrieval and interpretation

Beti Wyn Evans

Chapter 4 focuses on scenarios that require data retrieval and interpretation from at least one information source commonly found in pharmacies. Having identified from the scenario or situation what information you need to find, you are required to find the relevant information, and then solve the problem.

Before you embark on the following scenarios, make sure you are familiar with some key references used in everyday pharmacy practice. Take 5 minutes now to consider some of the key information sources used and list when you might use which resource.

Remember, many of these references are available online, but in an OSCE situation you may need to access the hard copy, so be familiar with the layout of both.

Key references

Baxter K, ed. (2010). *Stockley's Drug Interactions*, 9th edn. London: Pharmaceutical Press.
Joint Formulary Committee. *British National Formulary*. London: BMJ Group and Pharmaceutical Press.
Sweetman S, ed. (2011). *Martindale: the Complete Drug Reference*, 37th edn. Pharmaceutical Press.
Summaries of Product Characteristics
Patient Information Leaflets

In order to locate relevant information quickly and accurately you need to be familiar with the layout and content of the different reference sources. Familiarise yourself with the index, the sequence of chapters and the layout of information. Remember that information relating to one issue may appear in more than one place. For example, in the *BNF*, information about the side-effects of a medicine will appear under the drug details, but also potentially in the introductory section to the chapter in which the medicine is placed. Warnings from the Medicines and Healthcare Products Regulatory Agency about the safety of a medicine will typically appear in a shaded box within the general text in the introduction.

Learning objectives

The following OSCE scenarios assess data retrieval and interpretation skills. By the end of this chapter you should be able to:

- identify which reference source is the most appropriate to address which question
- retrieve information efficiently
- explain information in lay terms
- problem-solve.

Scenario 4.1 Identifying a foreign product and advice on monitoring

Format: Written station

Supporting material available to student: Copies of *Martindale* and *BNF*

Time allowed: 5 minutes

Suggested years of study: Undergraduate years 3, 4; pre-registration; postgraduate.

Knowledge and skills tested

- Identification of foreign medicines
- Data retrieval and interpretation
- Monitoring requirements.

Task

You are working in a community pharmacy when the local general practitioner telephones to ask you to identify medication taken by Mr T. Mr T has moved to the UK from New Zealand, and has just registered with the general practice in the UK.

Mr T takes atenolol 50 mg od, and Lipex® 40 mg od. The GP wishes to know:

1. What is Lipex®?
2. Is the dose of Lipex® within recommended limits? Explain your answer.
3. What laboratory parameters, if any, should be monitored in this patient?

Scenario 4.1 feedback

1. What is Lipex®?

Simvastatin. You should have used *Martindale* to find this information. *Martindale* is the best source of information for identifying trade names used worldwide. Do you need to practise finding this information?

2. Is the dose of Lipex® within recommended limits? Explain your answer

Yes, there are a number of different indications for simvastatin, however 40 mg daily is a reasonable dose for any of the indications. The most appropriate place to identify dosage information is the *BNF*.

3. What laboratory parameters, if any, should be monitored in this patient?

Answers should include lipid profile (total cholesterol and its constituents (HDL, LDL, TG)) as a measure of efficacy, and liver function tests (including the liver enzymes AST, ALT, and GGT (gamma glutamyltransferase)) to assess whether the statin can be safely prescribed. There may be occasions where the creatine kinase level should be monitored, if muscle damage is suspected. Note that the question asks for laboratory parameters, so no marks would be awarded for signs or symptoms.

Where would you find this information? The *BNF* does not generally contain complete information about monitoring. You would normally expect to find information about monitoring in guidelines, in Summaries of Product Characteristics and in texts which consider the therapeutic use of these drugs. Consider which sources are the most up to date. Some OSCE stations may test knowledge that you are expected to have at certain levels of study, not only what you can retrieve from a book.

Suggested revision points

- Monitoring requirements for lipid-regulating medication, and the components of lipid profiles and liver function tests
- Retrieval of information about monitoring from sources such as the *BNF*, SPCs (Summary of Product Characteristics), guidelines on the management of a condition (e.g. NICE).

Scenario 4.2 Excipients

Format: Written station

Supporting material available to student: *BNF*, copies of Patient Information Leaflets for more than one brand of paroxetine, to include Seroxat, and the Actavis UK Ltd. product

Time allowed: 5 minutes

Suggested years of study: Undergraduate years 3, 4; pre-registration; postgraduate.

Knowledge and skills tested

- Data retrieval and interpretation
- Problem-solving.

Task

One of your regular patients, Mrs DA, enters your pharmacy with a packet of paroxetine 30 mg tablets that you dispensed for her a week ago. She has responded well to paroxetine which she has been taking for severe depression for six months.

She has noticed that the tablets you have given her are not the same brand as the one she normally receives. She normally receives Seroxat®, but on this occasion she was dispensed a generic version made by Actavis UK Ltd.

In the last few days she has experienced a runny nose, and hives have appeared on her skin. She informs you that she is allergic to sunset yellow, and she asks you to check whether the tablets she has been dispensed contain this.

You need to address the following issues:

1. Answer Mrs DA's question – does the brand of tablets you have dispensed contain sunset yellow?
2. Offer an explanation to Mrs DA regarding the cause of her symptoms
3. Take action to resolve the problem – what will you do?
4. Establish what action you would take to prevent the problem from happening again.

Scenario 4.2 feedback

1. Answer Mrs DA's question – does the brand of tablets you have dispensed contain sunset yellow?

You are expected to make use of the material provided to you at the station, that is, the Patient Information Leaflets (PILs). An appropriate starting point would be the list of ingredients/additives/excipients in the PIL and/or Summary of Product Characteristics (SPCs) for paroxetine made by Actavis UK Ltd. If you read the list of ingredients you would have found that sunset yellow is an ingredient in the tablets you dispensed.

Note that the PIL or SPC is the most appropriate place to search for this kind of information. Both can be found online at www.medicines.org.uk (accessed 6 June 2012). SPCs and PILs follow a standard layout, which is useful to get to know so that you can locate information efficiently.

2. Offer an explanation to Mrs DA regarding the cause of her symptoms

Since the tablets dispensed contain sunset yellow, these may have caused the runny nose and hives. There may be other causes of her signs and symptoms, such as paroxetine itself, or another cause, unrelated to treatment.

At OSCE stations it is important to remember that there may be more than one answer to a question.

3. Take action to resolve the problem – what will you do?

Since you have been given more than one PIL at the OSCE station, you should check contents of other brands of paroxetine to establish whether they contain sunset yellow. You should then advise the use of a brand that does not contain sunset yellow.

4. Establish what action you would take to prevent the problem from happening again

Record the allergy to sunset yellow in the patient's medication record so that a future problem can be prevented. Advise Mrs

DA to tell the pharmacist of the allergy when receiving or purchasing new medication.

Suggested revision points

- Familiarity with the typical layout and content of PILs. The layout and subheadings used are the same for all PILs, regardless of the product.
- Use of patient medication records (PMRs) in community pharmacy.

Scenario 4.3 Contraception in nursing mothers

Format: Interactive station

Supporting material available to student: *BNF*

Time allowed: 5 minutes

Suggested years of study: Undergraduate year 4; pre-registration; postgraduate.

Knowledge and skills tested

- Asking the right questions
- Data retrieval and interpretation
- Communication.

Task

On a routine day in your pharmacy a female customer approaches you to ask what forms of oral contraception can be used when breastfeeding.

1. What questions do you ask? (Read the notes below after listing the questions you would ask.)

If you asked the appropriate questions you may be told that:

- the female customer is breastfeeding her newborn who is four weeks old
- she has been breastfeeding since delivery
- she is exclusively breastfeeding – no other milk has been given
- prior to her initial pregnancy she used a combined oral contraceptive (Microgynon® 30), which she would like to use again if possible.

2.   What advice do you give?

Scenario 4.3 feedback

1. What questions do you ask?

You should have:

- confirmed who is breastfeeding (Beware of jumping to conclusions, especially with customers who initiate a conversation with a general question such as 'What contraception do you recommend for breastfeeding mothers?')
- asked the age of the infant, because this determines whether oral contraception can be taken
- asked whether the breastfeeding mother is taking any other medication.

It would also be appropriate to ask about contraceptive history as this may indicate the woman's preferences for a particular contraceptive, and also any previous problems with contraceptives. Remember that the woman asked for advice regarding oral contraception, not any other method.

2. What advice do you give?

The *BNF* contains information about the forms of oral contraception available, and about their use in breastfeeding mothers.

Since the customer has indicated a preference for using a combined oral contraceptive, it is appropriate to first address whether this type of oral contraceptive can be taken.

Based on the information in the *BNF*, you should have advised that:

- combined oral contraception is inappropriate because of effects on lactation
- the alternative oral contraceptive is the progestogen-only pill (POP), which does not affect lactation
- POP can be started if the infant is older than three weeks. There is an increased risk of breakthrough bleeding if started earlier.

Suggested revision points

- Oral contraception options
- Contraception when breastfeeding.

Scenario 4.4 Vaccination advice

Format: Interactive station

Supporting material available to student: *BNF*

Time allowed: 5 minutes

Suggested years of study: Undergraduate year 4; pre-registration; postgraduate.

Knowledge and skills tested

- Communicating difficult issues
- Explaining benefit/risk issues in layperson terms.

Task

You are working as a community pharmacist when a male customer approaches you. He has been sent notification that his 12-month-old baby is scheduled to receive the first MMR (measles, mumps, rubella) vaccination in two weeks' time. He is concerned about the effects of the MMR vaccine, having read in the newspaper that there is a link with autism.

- How would you address the man's concerns?
- What advice and information would you offer?

Scenario 4.4 feedback

In this type of scenario, it is appropriate to acknowledge the man's concerns. That is, to show that you know there has been a lot of information in the media about this issue.

You should have then looked in the *BNF* for information relating to MMR. You should have identified a statement advising that there is no evidence of a link between MMR vaccination and autism. This is key in this scenario.

You should then have:

- explained the meaning of 'no evidence of a link', that is, it cannot be proven that the MMR vaccine causes autism
- discussed the benefits and risks of MMR vaccination, in terms of the consequences of the illnesses versus the possible side-effects of the vaccine. This might seem a lot to discuss in the short timeframe of the OSCE, so keep to main messages.

In interactive stations it is always sensible to check whether the person is satisfied with the information given. It is also important to avoid jargon and unexplained acronyms, that is, say things in lay language.

Suggested revision points

- Vaccination programmes for infants.

Scenario 4.5 Identifying a foreign product

Format: Written station

Supporting material available to student: *Martindale* and *BNF*

Time allowed: 5 minutes

Suggested years of study: Undergraduate years 1, 2.

Knowledge and skills tested

- Identification of medicines
- Data retrieval and interpretation.

Task

On your daily hospital ward round you meet a patient from Spain who is prescribed a drug called buformin. The drug is not available in the UK.

Answer the following questions:

1. To which group of drugs does buformin belong?
2. Which drug(s) of the same group are available in the UK?

Scenario 4.5 feedback

1. To which group of drugs does buformin belong?

Biguanides. You should have used *Martindale* to identify this. *Martindale* is the best source of information for identifying trade names used worldwide.

2. Which drug(s) of the same group are available in the UK?

Metformin. Having identified the group of drugs in *Martindale*, you should have then looked in the *BNF* to identify which biguanide is available in the UK.

Suggested revision points

- Locating brand names of products in *Martindale*.

Scenario 4.6 Intravenous drug administration

Format: Written station

Supporting material available to student: SPC for Bondronat® 2 mg and 6 mg concentrate for solution for infusion

Time allowed: 5 minutes

Suggested years of study: Undergraduate years 3, 4; pre-registration; postgraduate.

Knowledge and skills tested

- Data retrieval and interpretation
- Advice regarding intravenous administration of drugs.

Task

You are a hospital pharmacist working on a medical ward. The medical team has prescribed ibandronic acid intravenous infusion 2 mg stat for one of the patients, who has hypercalcaemia of malignancy. The nurse on duty has not given this drug before and would like some more information on how to administer it. The patient's albumin-corrected serum calcium is 3.2 mmol/L. The patient does not have renal or hepatic impairment.

You will need to refer to the Summary of Product Characteristics for Bondronat® 2 mg and 6 mg concentrate for solution for infusion to address the following questions:

1. Is the dose appropriate for this condition?
2. How much infusion fluid would you recommend that 2 mg is administered in?
3. List two infusion fluids that can be used to administer ibandronic acid.
4. Over what duration would you recommend that a dose of 2 mg be administered?

5. If the patient had a creatinine clearance of 34 mL/minute, and ibandronic acid was being used for the prevention of skeletal events in patients with breast cancer and metastatic bone disease, what is the recommended dosage and infusion duration?

Scenario 4.6 feedback

1. Is the dose appropriate for this condition?

No – the dose should be 4 mg as a single dose for this calcium level. You should have identified this information in the SPC.

Are you familiar with the layout and subheadings used in SPCs? If not, now is a good time to do this. Have a look at two different products at the same time to identify common aspects.

2. How much infusion fluid would you recommend that 2 mg is administered in?

500 mL (information from the SPC).

3. List two infusion fluids that can be used to administer ibandronic acid

Sodium chloride 0.9% or glucose 5% (information from the SPC).

4. Over what duration would you recommend that a dose of 2 mg be administered?

2 hours (information from the SPC).

5. If the patient had a creatinine clearance of 34 mL/minute, and ibandronic acid was being used for the prevention of skeletal events in patients with breast cancer and metastatic bone disease, what is the recommended dosage and infusion duration?

4 mg over 1 hour. Did you locate the table providing this information in the SPC? Which section? (Note that you are only given the SPC as a source of information for this scenario.)

Suggested revision points

■ Layout and content of SPCs, with particular reference to dosage information and advice about administration.

Chapter 4 feedback summary

In Chapter 4 you have looked at some key reference sources used to deal with day-to-day enquiries in pharmacy, including the *BNF*, SPCs, PILs and *Martindale*. The use of *Stockley's Drug Interactions* is considered in Chapter 5.

In this chapter you have learned that knowing your way around book indexes, and being familiar with layout of information is key to efficient retrieval of information. You have practised finding information from several sources used in everyday practice, and have applied that information to case scenarios.

Now that you have completed this chapter, assess your competence in the knowledge and skills listed in Table 4.1. Jot down any notes that may help you.

Table 4.1   Chapter 4 learning outcomes

Knowledge and skills	More work required	Feel competent
Identify which reference source is the most appropriate to address which question		
Retrieve information efficiently		
Explain information in lay terms		
Problem-solve		

If there are any points that you consider need further work, start a CPD (continuous professional development) cycle now to identify how you can achieve this action.

References and further reading

Baxter K, ed. (2010). *Stockley's Drug Interactions,* 9th edn. London: Pharmaceutical Press.

British National Formulary available from http://www.bnf.org/bnf/index.htm (accessed 11 June 2012).

Patient Information Leaflets from www.medicines.org.uk/emc (accessed 11 June 2012).

Summaries of Product Characteristics from www.medicines.org.uk/emc (accessed 11 June 2012).

Sweetman S, ed. (2011) *Martindale: the Complete Drug Reference,* 37th edn. London: Pharmaceutical Press.

5

Clinical prescription management problems

Laura Kravitz and Aamer Safdar

Chapter 5 is focused on problem-solving around everyday prescription issues such as drug interactions; the selection of appropriate treatment; drug monitoring and choice of treatment in patients with a chronic condition. You will be asked to apply your knowledge of medicines to clinical practice.

Within an OSCE scenario it is important to identify the most appropriate source of information quickly, retrieve the information and apply it to the patient's prescription. Chapter 5 applies the material covered in Chapter 4 on data retrieval and interpretation.

Before attempting the scenarios in Chapter 5 you should revise your notes on the management of common conditions.

Take 5 minutes now to consider some of the key information resources used in everyday practice and list when you might use which resource. Many of these resources are available online.

Key references

Baxter K, ed. (2010). *Stockley's Drug Interactions*, 9th edn. London: Pharmaceutical Press.

Joint Formulary Committee. *British National Formulary*. London: BMJ Group and Pharmaceutical Press.

Sweetman S, ed. (2011). *Martindale: the Complete Drug Reference*, 37th edn. Pharmaceutical Press.

Summaries of Product Characteristics

Patient Information Leaflets

You can see that these references are the same as those listed in Chapter 4. This is because this chapter focuses on clinical application.

Learning objectives

The following scenarios assess clinical problem-solving skills. By the end of this chapter you should be able to:

- review prescriptions and identify clinical management problems
- choose appropriate reference materials in order to answer the questions
- retrieve appropriate material in order to solve the problem(s) identified
- interpret laboratory data
- apply information to the scenario
- communicate recommendations and advice to patients and prescribers.

For each of the following scenarios, remember to read the scenarios fully and think about the topic before you consider tackling the issue.

Scenario 5.1 Managing interactions (hyperkalaemia)

Format: Written station

Supporting material available to student: *BNF*

Time allowed: 5 minutes

Suggested years of study: Undergraduate years 3, 4; pre-registration.

Knowledge and skills tested

- Prescription management and interpretation of data
- Problem-solving.

Task

As a hospital pharmacist you are making your daily visit to a medical ward. You are given a prescription to prepare for Mr S to go home. Mr S was taking co-amilozide before coming in to hospital, for water retention. He has since been started on lisinopril to treat heart failure. His serum potassium level is 5.4 mmol/L, which has increased from 4.3 mmol/L on admission to hospital. (Normal potassium range 3.5–5.0 mmol/L.)

His prescription for taking home is:

- co-amilozide 5/50 mg i mane
- lisinopril 20 mg i mane.

1. Is this prescription clinically appropriate? Explain your answer
2. What action(s) would you recommend? Explain your answer.

Scenario 5.1 feedback

1. Is this prescription clinically appropriate? Explain your answer

No, there is an interaction between co-amilozide and lisinopril. Co-amilozide is a combination of a thiazide diuretic (hydrochlorothiazide) and a potassium-sparing diuretic (amiloride) which leads to potassium retention. ACE inhibitors also cause potassium retention, therefore there is a risk of hyperkalaemia. From the laboratory results it is clear that there is evidence of the interaction, with the potassium level already exceeding the upper limit of normal.

2. What action(s) would you recommend? Explain your answer

What are the guidelines for the treatment of heart failure? When an interaction is identified you need to decide which medicine, if any, to adjust or change. Here, both drugs are recommended for heart failure. In addition the patient is retaining fluid. You know that ACE inhibitors may cause hyperkalaemia, so the most sensible option is *not* to use a potassium-sparing diuretic. The best solution here is to choose a loop diuretic only, such as furosemide in place of co-amilozide.

It is important that you mention how to monitor whether your suggestions have solved the clinical problem. Here you would recommend that serum potassium levels are monitored. Many students lose marks in OSCEs by failing to follow-up recommendations suggested. Your solution can only be considered successful if the patient recovers!

You need to be familiar with Appendix 1 of the *BNF* (Interactions), especially the subheadings. Here you needed to know that co-amilozide is a combination of amiloride and hydrochlorothiazide (and what type of diuretic each of these is) in order to search for an interaction with lisinopril, an ACE inhibitor.

You are not expected to know all guidelines! Brief summaries for many conditions are found in the *BNF*.

Suggested revision points

- Mechanism of potassium-sparing effects of ACE inhibitors
- Heart failure management
- Patient monitoring.

Scenario 5.2 Advising how to use lamotrigine

Format: Written or interactive station

Supporting material available to student: *BNF*

Time allowed: 5 minutes

Suggested years of study: Undergraduate years 2–4; pre-registration; postgraduate.

Knowledge and skills tested

- Data retrieval and interpretation
- Providing advice to a GP
- Application of information to the patient scenario.

Task

You are working as a pharmacist in a hospital medicines information department when a GP calls for advice regarding initiating lamotrigine tablets for a 40-year-old female patient with a diagnosis of epilepsy. The GP is on a home visit, has no access to a *BNF* and cannot remember the dose for lamotrigine. The patient is currently taking sodium valproate tablets 600 mg twice daily.

1. What is lamotrigine used for in this patient?
2. How should lamotrigine be initiated?
3. Suggest a typical maintenance dose of lamotrigine
4. What other essential information would you give the GP (and patient)?

Scenario 5.2 feedback

1. What is lamotrigine used for in this patient?

Lamotrigine is used as monotherapy and adjunctive treatment of focal seizures and generalised seizures, including tonic-clonic seizures. Use the terminology in the *BNF* to answer this type of question, it is easy to lose marks.

2. How should lamotrigine be initiated?

Here you should advise on dosage titration, including time intervals. Specific dosage information should be given. Drugs used for the treatment of some conditions, such as epilepsy, are also used for a number of other indications (not all licensed). You must be careful when using the *BNF* index to select the correct indication – dosages may vary. Do not 'reinterpret' this information – read it as it is. It is so easy to lose marks here too!

3. Suggest a typical maintenance dose of lamotrigine

Usual maintenance, 100–200 mg daily in 1–2 divided doses.

4. What other essential information would you give the GP (and patient)?

The *BNF* lists two cautions/warnings for lamotrigine. Both must be communicated with the GP/patient:

- Patients should be alert for symptoms and signs that may suggest bone marrow failure, such as anaemia, bruising or infection. This is because aplastic anaemia, bone marrow depression and pancytopenia have been associated rarely with lamotrigine.
- Look out for a rash, particularly in the first eight weeks of treatment. Serious skin reactions including Stevens–Johnson syndrome and toxic epidermal necrolysis (rarely with fatalities) have developed, especially in children. Rash is sometimes associated with hypersensitivity syndrome and is more common in patients with history of allergy or rash from other antiepileptic drugs. Consider withdrawal if rash or signs of hypersensitivity syndrome develop. Factors associated with increased risk of serious skin reactions include concomitant use of valproate, higher initial lamotrigine dosing and more rapid dose escalation than is recommended.

Suggested revision points

- Have a look at classification in epilepsy, this has a significant impact on choice of treatment
- Remind yourself of the impact of liver enzyme induction/ inhibition on treatment choice.

Scenario 5.3 Managing interactions (St John's Wort)

Format: Written or interactive station

Supporting material available to student: *BNF, Stockley's Drug Interactions*

Time allowed: 5 minutes

Suggested years of study: Undergraduate years 2–4; pre-registration; postgraduate.

Knowledge and skills tested

- Data retrieval and interpretation
- Providing advice to a GP
- Application of information to the patient scenario.

Task

An elderly patient wishes to speak to you about their cough and wheeze, which they have experienced for a few days now. The cough is 'dry' and as they have been feeling wheezy, they have needed to use their asthma inhalers more often than usual over the last few days. When asked about medication, the patient states that apart from the inhalers, he takes Uniphyllin Continus® (for the last year), his dose having gone up to 400 mg every 12 hours last month. Also for the last three months he has been taking St John's Wort, as he has been feeling 'low' since a friend passed away, although that is not a medicine but something 'natural' he states.

1. What is the most likely cause of the patient's symptoms?
2. What mechanism of interaction could be involved here, and what are the consequences of the interaction?
3. Should the patient just stop taking the St John's Wort? Explain your answer.

Scenario 5.3 feedback

1. What is the most likely cause of the patient's symptoms?

There is an interaction between theophylline (Uniphyllin Continus®) and St John's Wort. This results in a reduction in plasma concentration of theophylline, allowing symptoms of asthma to reappear/break through. That is, the lower plasma level of theophylline is not controlling asthma/breathing.

2. What mechanism of interaction could be involved here, and what are the consequences of the interaction?

St John's Wort is an enzyme inducer, resulting in increased theophylline metabolism and consequently reduced plasma concentration of theophylline. This lower plasma theophylline level is insufficient to control the patient's symptoms.

Note each stage of the answer to part 2. Students frequently lose marks by missing a stage of the explanation. Read questions carefully and make sure you address each element.

3. Should the patient just stop taking the St John's Wort? Explain your answer

No, the patient should contact his GP in order to manage this clinical situation. There is potential for withdrawal symptoms from St John's Wort and toxicity from raised theophylline levels if St John's Wort is stopped suddenly.

The patient's theophylline levels need to be monitored. (The usual interval is 5 days after adjusting treatment, the plasma level being taken 4–6 hours post dose.)

As with Scenario 5.1, it is easy to lose marks by not mentioning how you will monitor the patient's response to treatment adjustment.

Did you use the *BNF* to answer this question? Could you answer all parts of the question using the *BNF*? The *BNF* provides basic information on drug interactions. More detailed information is available in *Stockley's Drug Interactions*. You can save time in an OSCE by using this text first, if it is provided.

Suggested revision points

- Make a list of drugs with narrow therapeutic indices, these are the most likely to be affected by the addition of an enzyme inducer/inhibitor
- Identify the drugs that are monitored by measuring serum levels – there are not very many!

Scenario 5.4 Choosing antibiotic therapy

Format: Written or interactive station

Supporting material available to student: *BNF*

Time allowed: 5 minutes

Suggested years of study: Undergraduate year 4, pre-registration, postgraduate.

Knowledge and skills tested

- Signs and symptoms of penicillin allergy
- Decision-making.

Task

On your daily ward visit you are approached by a junior doctor who asks about suitability of therapy for a 5-year-old child who has been diagnosed with meningitis thought to be caused by meningococci. Lumbar puncture cultures have been taken and the infection is sensitive to benzylpenicillin, which the doctor would like to prescribe. Other microbial sensitivities are not yet known.

The child's medicine chart notes that the patient is allergic to penicillin. The nature of the allergy is documented as 'rash (more than 72 hours after previous administration), no sign of anaphylaxis'.

1. Which antibiotic therapy would you recommend for the patient?
2. Why would you recommend this choice? Explain your answer with reference to the information you have been given.
3. What advice would you give to the nursing staff about monitoring this patient with reference to allergic reactions?

Scenario 5.4 feedback

1. Which antibiotic therapy would you recommend for the patient?

Benzylpenicillin can be given to this patient, although it is a penicillin antibiotic. You can find information about which antibacterials are recommended for which infection in the *BNF*.

2. Why would you recommend this choice? Explain your answer with reference to the information you have been given

It is easy to make decisions based on 'the patient is allergic, find something else'. This is the type of case that demonstrates the role of the pharmacist in a clinical team. This patient is seriously ill, with a life-threatening condition. At this stage the only antibiotic that you *know* to be effective is benzylpenicillin. A rash that develops more than 72 hours after previous administration does not constitute an allergic reaction. Your professional judgement should lead you to the conclusion that the risk associated with not starting treatment with the penicillin antibiotic (as soon as possible) outweighs the benefits of avoiding the drug because of worries around allergy.

3. What advice would you give to the nursing staff about monitoring this patient with reference to allergic reactions?

Nursing staff should monitor for signs of worsening allergy, such as early rash or anaphylaxis. Adrenaline should be available on the ward, with information on administration readily available to nursing and medical staff.

Did you use the *BNF* to answer this question? Could you answer all parts of the question using the *BNF*? You might need to refer to the *BNF for Children* to confirm information on paediatric dosage.

Suggested revision points

- Be certain that you know the definitions of the terms 'allergy' and 'sensitivity'. Many students confuse the two terms
- Antibacterial treatment options for different infections.

Scenario 5.5 Managing interactions (ibuprofen)

Format: Written or interactive station

Supporting material available to student: *BNF*; *Stockley's Drug Interactions*

Time allowed: 5 minutes

Suggested years of study: Undergraduate years 2–4; pre-registration; postgraduate.

Knowledge and skills tested

- Data retrieval and interpretation
- Knowledge of reference sources
- Identification of clinical problems
- Problem-solving.

Task

You are working in your community pharmacy and are approached by Mr P, a 40-year-old man with a history of depression. Your records show that he is currently prescribed sertraline 100 mg daily. He has hurt his back while playing rugby. One of his friends has suggested ibuprofen 200 mg tablets, which helped him when similarly injured. He asks your advice about dosage.

What advice will you give Mr P?

Scenario 5.5 feedback

Mr P is currently prescribed sertraline to treat depression. This is a selective serotonin reuptake inhibitor (SSRI) antidepressant. Ibuprofen is a non-steroidal anti-inflammatory drug (NSAID). There is an increased risk of bleeding when NSAIDs are given with SSRIs ('black dot' interaction).

Mr P should be advised not to take ibuprofen.

Of course Mr P still has a bad back! At this point you should ask questions in order to determine the severity of pain. Then you could recommend paracetamol 1 g q.d.s. or co-codamol 8/500 mg, two tablets/capsules q.d.s.

Did you use the *BNF* to answer this? *BNF* Appendix 1 is a quick and easy source of interaction information (*Stockley's Drug Interactions* provides more detailed information). Using Appendix 1 is often dependent on knowing the class of a drug, for example that sertraline is an SSRI. If you look up the drug in the *BNF* index and find the main citation, this lists drugs according to the classification.

Remember you must ask customers/patients questions about other medicines. In this type of scenario, where information about prescribed medicines is given, students frequently forget to ask about over-the-counter (OTC) medicines.

Suggested revision points

- Some medicines, such as NSAIDs, lithium, erythromycin, warfarin and carbamazepine, are frequently implicated in interaction scenarios. Familiarise yourself with these drugs and look at the mechanism(s) of the interaction(s). This will enable you to identify these interactions more easily.

Scenario 5.6 Initiating warfarin therapy

Format: Interactive station

Supporting information available to student: *BNF*, information on loading regimens (depending on year of study)

Time allowed: 5 minutes

Suggested years of study: Undergraduate years 3, 4; pre-registration; postgraduate.

Knowledge and skills tested

- Anticoagulation regimens
- Use of warfarin
- Common drug interactions.

Task

A junior doctor has called you for advice regarding a male patient, aged 50 years, for whom the consultant has requested warfarin be started. The patient has had a mechanical mitral valve replacement inserted and requires anticoagulation. His past medical history includes hypertension, type 2 diabetes and ischaemic heart disease. He has no known drug allergies and none of his medicines interacts with warfarin.

1. What dose would you recommend for initiation of warfarin?
2. What INR range would you recommend and why?
3. What maintenance dose would you recommend?

Scenario 5.6 feedback

1. What dose would you recommend for initiation of warfarin?

There are a number of different warfarin loading dose regimens, ranging from 10 mg, 10 mg, 5 mg on days 1, 2, 3 (Fennerty *et al.*, 1988) to 5 mg, 5 mg, 5 mg (Tait and Sefcick, 1998; Crowther *et al.*, 1997, 1999). The key is to ensure the INR is tested on day 3 and the warfarin dose adjusted accordingly.

2. What INR range would you recommend and why?

The recommended INR range is 2.5–4.5 depending on local guidelines, the number of mechanical heart valves and other patient risk factors. The higher INR is because mechanical mitral valves have a higher risk of clotting so therefore require more anticoagulation.

3. What maintenance dose would you recommend?

The maintenance dose of warfarin is dependent on the INR and, in this scenario, it would be unwise to recommend a specific warfarin dose. There are a number of nomograms and local guidelines for adjusting doses of warfarin. Patients have different sensitivities to warfarin so one patient may require a much higher dose of warfarin to achieve the same INR as another patient. There are also a number of drug interactions and foods that may affect the INR.

Suggested revision points

- Review your local warfarin guidelines and identify the different loading regimens
- From the guidelines, list the different conditions that require warfarin anticoagulation and their corresponding INR ranges
- List the drugs that interact with warfarin and identify whether the INR would be increased or decreased.

Scenario 5.7 Drug-induced hypercalcaemia

Format: Written station

Supporting material available to student: *BNF* and SPC for One-Alpha® capsules

Time allowed: 5 minutes

Suggested years of study: Undergraduate year 4; pre-registration; postgraduate.

Knowledge and skills tested

- Identification and management of drug-induced problems
- Interpretation of laboratory data
- Problem-solving.

Task

On your daily hospital ward visit you come across a patient who has been admitted because of severe nausea and vomiting. The patient has hypertension and hypoparathyroidism. His current medication is bendroflumethiazide 2.5 mg in the morning and One-Alpha® 1 microgram daily. The laboratory test results shown in Table 5.1 have just been returned to the ward.

Answer the following questions:

1. Comment on the laboratory test results, identifying any that are of concern.
2. What might be the cause of any observations you made in response to question 1?
3. What action(s) would you recommend?

Table 5.1 Laboratory results for Scenario 5.7

Test (normal range)	Result
Sodium (137–145 mmol/L)	139
Potassium (3.6–5.0 mmol/L)	4.8
Calcium (2.15–2.65 mmol/L)	2.9
Phosphate (0.8–1.4 mmol/L)	1.3

Scenario 5.7 feedback

1. Comment on the laboratory test results, identifying any that are of concern

The calcium level is raised, that is, higher than the upper limit of the normal range.

2. What might be the cause of any observations you made in response to question 1?

There are two potential causes:

- the bendroflumethiazide, a thiazide diuretic, may increase the risk of hypercalcaemia
- alfacalcidol (One-Alpha®), being converted to 1,25-dihydroxyvitamin D (which regulates calcium metabolism), results in increased absorption of calcium. Since hypercalcaemia is observed, it is possible that the dose of alfacalcidol is too high.

3. What action(s) would you recommend?

Stop One-Alpha® treatment until the plasma calcium concentration returns to normal. Then restart alfacalcidol at half the dose, which is 0.5 microgram daily in this patient. In addition, calcium levels should be monitored.

Many students panic when they encounter a term with which they are unfamiliar, such as in this case hypoparathyroidism. Here the term is used to explain the need for One-Alpha®. You will not be expected to know every clinical condition!

Which resource did you use to help you answer the questions? Some relevant information is available in the *BNF*, but may be time consuming to find. You will need to look in the side-effects section in the classification part of the citation. If you are given an SPC for One-Alpha® the information is more easily found, and is particularly useful for what to recommend if hypercalcaemia occurs during treatment. You can practise looking at SPCs (and Patient Information Leaflets – PILs) at www.medicines.org.uk/emc/ (accessed 6 June 2012).

Suggested revision points

Practise looking at SPCs and PILs, so that you do not waste time looking to find where specific information is located.

Are you familiar with the terminology such as hypo/ hyperkalaemia, hypo/hypernatraemia? If not, revise these terms, which are used frequently.

Scenario 5.8 Drug choice in nursing mothers

Format: Interactive station

Supporting material available to student: *BNF*

Time allowed: 5 minutes

Suggested years of study: Undergraduate years 3, 4; pre-registration; postgraduate.

Knowledge and skills tested

- Data retrieval and interpretation
- Knowledge of reference sources
- Identification of clinical problems
- Problem-solving.

Task

Mrs C, a patient who is known to you, attends the pharmacy wishing to purchase ibuprofen 400 mg t.d.s. to treat back pain. Mrs C gave birth two months ago.

1. What questions do you need to ask Mrs C?
2. What advice would you offer Mrs C?

Scenario 5.8 feedback

1. What questions do you need to ask Mrs C?

In addition to the standard WWHAM (remind yourself of what this is – see Chapter 1), you need to ask Mrs C if she is breastfeeding.

2. What advice would you offer Mrs C?

The *BNF* states that the amount of ibuprofen secreted into breast milk is too small to be harmful. Nevertheless, some manufacturers advise avoiding ibuprofen, including topical application, while breastfeeding.

If you choose to advise that Mrs C does not take ibuprofen, you need to suggest an alternative analgesic. Paracetamol is considered safe in breastfeeding.

This scenario requires you to retrieve a single piece of information. Many of the marks available will be for how you communicate the information to the patient.

A more complex OSCE may require you to make a decision about a medicine for which there is no obvious alternative, or perhaps a condition which is more life threatening. In these situations, you may have to consider suggesting that the mother discontinues breastfeeding, particularly if there is little published evidence that breastfeeding is safe while taking a particular medicine. Alternatively it may be advisable for the mother to express breast milk and discard for the duration of treatment, then continue once treatment is no longer required.

Did you use the *BNF* to answer this? The information required to answer this question is available in the *BNF*. The SPC also contains information about pregnancy and breast-feeding.

Suggested revision points

- Familiarise yourself with your *BNF*. Where can you find information about breastfeeding, pregnancy and use of drugs in hepatic or renal failure?

Scenario 5.9 Managing interactions (warfarin)

Format: Written or interactive station

Supporting material available to student: *BNF*, *Stockley's Drug Interactions*

Time allowed: 5 minutes

Suggested years of study: Undergraduate years 3,4; pre-registration; postgraduate.

Knowledge and skills tested

- Data retrieval and interpretation
- Knowledge of reference sources
- Identification of clinical problems
- Problem-solving.

Task

You are a hospital pharmacist. A junior doctor is asking your advice. Ideally she would like to prescribe clarithromycin for one of her patients, however the patient takes warfarin. The junior doctor is aware of the interaction between clarithromycin and warfarin and would like your opinion on whether treatment could be initiated.

What is your advice?

Scenario 5.9 feedback

How did you approach this type of scenario? First, you need to find out about the details of the interaction between the two drugs. Does the interaction mean that you cannot use the two drugs together? If you do use the drugs together what, if any, monitoring may be required?

Clarithromycin interacts with warfarin, which increases the anticoagulant effect. The importance is established and potentially serious. The mechanism of action is inhibition of the liver enzymes CYP450. This reduces clearance of warfarin, resulting in increased levels of warfarin in the blood, resulting in an increase in the INR, and an increased risk of bleeding.

Clarithromycin can be taken by patients on warfarin if it is the most appropriate treatment, but the INR must be monitored closely. You need to identify through discussion with the prescriber whether clarithromycin is the most appropriate treatment in this case, or whether there is a safer alternative. If clarithromycin is to be prescribed, you need to offer advice on managing the interaction.

Remember that OSCEs assess your ability to communicate appropriately. Here you are responding to another healthcare professional, so language and detail must reflect this. It would be inappropriate (and you would lose marks) to simply respond saying 'there is an interaction'. You would be expected to offer a solution. In this case you would recommend initiating treatment and monitoring to reduce risk.

- Did you use the *BNF* to answer this question?
- Could you answer the question in enough detail using the *BNF*?

This scenario clearly demonstrates the importance of choosing the most appropriate source of information. *BNF* Appendix 1 gives insufficient information to answer this question in detail; *Stockley's Drug Interactions* is the most appropriate reference source here.

Suggested revision points

- Are you confident on the use of prothrombin times? What does a raised INR mean? What does an INR of 2 mean, and how would you explain this to a patient?

Scenario 5.10 Clopidogrel for percutaneous coronary intervention

Format: Written station

Supporting information available to student: *BNF*

Time allowed: 5 minutes

Suggested years of study: Pre-registration; postgraduate.

Knowledge and skills tested

- Interventional cardiology
- Percutaneous coronary intervention (PCI) stent types
- Antiplatelet therapy.

Task

You are in the dispensary and receive a call from a local GP who has a hospital referral letter for a 60-year-old woman which recommends prescribing clopidogrel 75 mg to be taken daily. The patient was admitted to hospital for a PCI and had a stent inserted. The GP is unsure how long the treatment with clopidogrel should be continued for and wants your advice.

1. What types of stents are routinely used in hospitals?
2. How does the type of stent affect the length of treatment?
3. What length of course is appropriate for each type of stent?

Scenario 5.10 feedback

1. What types of stents are routinely used in hospitals?

The first thing you will need to find out from either the GP or the hospital is the type of stent that the patient has had inserted. The common stents are either 'bare metal stents' or 'drug-eluting stents'. Post-procedural management of patients with coronary stents is focused on prevention of stent thrombosis and secondary prevention of the underlying vascular disease.

2. How does the type of stent affect the length of treatment?

3. What length of course is appropriate for each type of stent?

The duration of clopidogrel therapy is determined by the clinical setting. Patients whose stents – bare metal stents or drug-eluting stents – were implanted for a non-ST elevation myocardial infarction should be treated for 12 months. Patients with stable angina treated with a bare metal stent should take clopidogrel for at least one month and patients receiving a drug-eluting stent should continue clopidogrel therapy for 6–12 months.

Suggested revision points

- Guidance on PCI and use of stents and antiplatelet therapy
- Identify the types of stents commonly used and patient risk factors in terms of when to use them.

Scenario 5.11 Managing therapy (ciprofloxacin)

Format: Interactive station

Supporting information available to student: *BNF*

Time allowed: 5 minutes

Suggested years of study: Undergraduate years 3, 4; pre-registration; postgraduate.

Knowledge and skills tested

- Antibiotics and their indications
- Drug interactions
- Patient counselling.

Task

You are in a community pharmacy and receive a prescription for a 65-year-old male patient for ciprofloxacin 500 mg to be taken twice daily for seven days. You note from his patient medication record (PMR) that the patient has previously had numerous courses of trimethoprim. You also note that the patient currently takes the following medicines:

- Aspirin 75 mg daily
- Rampiril 5 mg daily
- Simvastatin 40 mg daily
- Sodium valproate (Epilim Chrono®) 300 mg daily.

He has no known drug allergies.

1. What is the likely indication for the ciprofloxacin?
2. Which, if any, of his medicines may interfere with ciprofloxacin?
3. What counselling points are important for this patient?
4. What discussion might you want to have with the patient or his doctor?

Scenario 5.11 feedback

1. What is the likely indication for the ciprofloxacin?

There are a number of indications for ciprofloxacin but in this case it is most likely to be urinary tract infections (UTIs); the use of trimethoprim provides a clue that the patient may be experiencing recurrent UTIs.

2. Which, if any, of his medicines may interfere with ciprofloxacin?

There are no direct drug–drug interactions with ciprofloxacin for this patient.

3. What counselling points are important for this patient?

Specific counselling points for patients who are prescribed ciprofloxacin are that the medicine may impair performance of skilled tasks (e.g. driving), and that the effects are enhanced by alcohol.

4. What discussion might you want to have with the patient or his doctor?

Patients with epilepsy should be advised to use ciprofloxacin with caution because there is a risk that the seizure threshold may be reduced. Any decision needs to be discussed with the patient and ciprofloxacin used after weighing up the risks and benefits to the patient.

The *BNF* advises that tendon damage, including rupture, has been reported with quinolones. Tendon rupture may occur within 48 hours of starting treatment, although some cases have been reported months after stopping a quinolone. Quinolones are contraindicated in patients with a history of tendon disorders related to quinolone use. Prescribers should also be reminded that patients over 60 years of age are more prone to tendon damage; the risk of tendon damage is increased by the concomitant use of corticosteroids; and that if tendinitis is suspected, the quinolone should be discontinued immediately.

Suggested revision points

- List the common drug interactions with ciprofloxacin
- List the important counselling points, paying particular attention to any *BNF* warnings/advice.

Scenario 5.12 Ibuprofen in asthma

Format: Interactive station

Supporting information available to student: *BNF*

Time allowed: 5 minutes

Suggested years of study: Undergraduate years 3, 4; pre-registration; postgraduate.

Knowledge and skills tested

- Pain relief
- Management of drug–patient interactions.

Task

A young female patient comes into your pharmacy and wants to buy over-the-counter ibuprofen for her headache. You know this patient well and know that she suffers from moderate asthma and has inhalers for this condition. Your counter assistant is about to make the sale after having established the need for the medicine but does not consult with you. You know that the patient is known to be allergic to aspirin.

   The patient is prescribed the following medicines:

- salbutamol 100 microgram metered dose inhaler (MDI), two puffs four times a day when required
- Seretide® 250/50 MDI, two puffs twice daily
- theophylline modified release (Uniphyllin Continus®) 400 mg twice daily.

   What would be your advice to the patient and why?

Scenario 5.12 feedback

If the patient is allergic to aspirin, it is important to establish the nature of the allergy. If it is a 'true' allergy which results in anaphylaxis-type reactions (e.g. lip and throat swelling) then she may have similar reactions with other NSAIDs. There is a risk that if the patient is allergic she may suffer from bronchospasm, which would result in a worsening of her asthma. In this case ibuprofen may not be an appropriate choice. Simple analgesics such as paracetamol-based preparations would be a good first choice to start with.

Suggested revision points

- Identify the mechanism of action of NSAIDs
- Identify how NSAIDs may result in bronchospasm
- List the drugs that may be appropriate for this patient.

Scenario 5.13 Managing tuberculosis treatment regimens

Format: Interactive station

Supporting information available to student: *BNF*

Time allowed: 5 minutes

Suggested years of study: Undergraduate years 3, 4; pre-registration; postgraduate.

Knowledge and skills tested

- Infectious diseases
- Treatment regimens for tuberculosis.

Task

A 45-year-old African patient who has been taking treatment for tuberculosis for two months comes to the hospital pharmacy with the following repeat prescription. He weighs 60 kg.

The prescribed items are:

- Rifater® 6 tablets daily
- Ethambutol 1100 mg daily.

1. Why would you not be able to dispense the prescription?
2. What information will you need from the patient?
3. What recommendation will you make to the prescriber?

Scenario 5.13 feedback

1. Why would you not be able to dispense the prescription?

The first thing to do in this scenario is to identify from the *BNF* which regimen the patient is currently prescribed. He appears to be taking the recommended dosage for 'standard unsupervised six-month treatment'.

The regimen listed in the scenario is for the initial two months period only and needs to be changed for the next four months.

2. What information will you need from the patient?

The doses of the medicines are based on the patient's weight so it is important that these are adjusted accordingly. The initial doses are based on the patient weighing over 70 kg and his weight seems to have dropped by more than 10 kg over the last two months.

The patient's weight needs to be confirmed in order to prescribe appropriate dosages of drugs for the four-month continuation phase.

3. What recommendation will you make to the prescriber?

The four-month continuation phase of treatment should include two drugs only – that is, rifampicin and isoniazid. If the patient's weight is confirmed as being over 50 kg, the treatment recommended is 2 tablets daily of Rifinah® 300/150.

If combination products are not appropriate, dosage information for individual drugs is given in the *BNF*.

Suggested revision points

- Antituberculosis treatment regimens (*BNF* section).

Scenario 5.14 Antibiotic therapy in pregnancy

Format: Interactive station

Supporting information available to student: *BNF*

Time allowed: 5 minutes

Suggested years of study: Undergraduate years 3, 4; pre-registration; postgraduate.

Knowledge and skills tested

- Antibiotic use in pregnancy
- Patient counselling.

Task

You are in a community pharmacy and receive a prescription for a 35-year-old female patient for ciprofloxacin 500 mg to be taken twice daily for seven days. You note from her PMR that the patient was previously taking the combined oral contraceptive pill (Microgynon®) but did not get her repeat prescription for this the last time it was due. She is currently taking folic acid 400 micrograms daily which she recently purchased from your pharmacy. She has no known drug allergies.

1. What is the likely indication for the ciprofloxacin?
2. What information will you need from the patient to ensure the appropriateness of this prescription?

3. If the prescription is inappropriate, what would be your recommendation?

Scenario 5.14 feedback

1. What is the likely indication for the ciprofloxacin?

There are a number of indications for ciprofloxacin but in this case it is most likely to be urinary tract infections (UTIs), although you cannot be sure without asking the patient.

2. What information will you need from the patient to ensure the appropriateness of this prescription?

The clue in the question is that the patient may have stopped taking the combined oral contraceptive pill and she has recently purchased folic acid. The dose of folic acid indicates that she may be intending to get pregnant or may indeed be pregnant. The choice of antibiotic is therefore important depending on the stage of pregnancy, known as the trimester, which she is currently in.

Do you know where to locate information about drugs in pregnancy within the *BNF*?

3. If the prescription is inappropriate, what would be your recommendation?

The patient should be referred back to the GP for a new prescription of an antibiotic that can be taken in pregnancy. You should communicate this sensitively to the patient with reassurance that alternative options are available for use in pregnancy.

Suggested revision points

- List the antibiotics which are contraindicated for use in pregnancy
- Identify whether the trimester is important for the contraindication.

Chapter 5 feedback summary

In Chapter 5 you have looked at a range of clinical prescription management issues. Working through the scenarios should have enabled you to develop your prescription management and problem-solving skills.

Remember that when reviewing a prescription:

- You need to consider whether there is an actual or potential problem in relation to drug therapy. Don't forget about drug–disease interactions as well as drug–drug interactions. Look for evidence of a problem in the scenario and/or through talking to the patient or healthcare professional (e.g. signs or symptoms, adverse changes in laboratory data).
- It is important to consider the options available to solve the problem.
- You should recommend an appropriate solution to the problem, using the appropriate reference sources, and the information from the scenario. That is, the advice you give should be tailored to the given circumstances. Don't forget that recommendations may include advice on monitoring to ensure treatment is safe and/or effective.

In an OSCE station you should expect to explain (justify) your chosen course of action. Use the most appropriate reference sources available to you. When giving advice or recommendations to patients or healthcare professionals make sure you are communicating that advice clearly in a logical order, using language that is appropriate to the person you are talking to.

Now that you have completed this chapter, assess your competence in the knowledge and skills listed in Table 5.2. Jot down any notes that may help you.

If there are any points that you consider need further work, start a CPD (continuous professional development) cycle now to identify how you can achieve this action.

Table 5.2 Chapter 5 learning outcomes

Knowledge and skills	More work required	Feel competent
Review prescriptions and identify clinical management problems		
Choose appropriate reference materials in order to answer the questions		
Retrieve appropriate material in order to solve the problem(s) identified		
Interpret laboratory data		
Apply information to the scenario		
Communicate recommendations and advice to patients and prescribers		

References and further reading

Baxter K, ed. (2010). *Stockley's Drug Interactions*, 9th edn. London: Pharmaceutical Press.

Crowther MA, Harrison L, Hirsch J (1997). Reply: warfarin: less may be better. *Arch Intern Med* 127: 332–333.

Crowther MA, Ginsberg JB, Kearon C *et al.* (1999). A randomized trial comparing 5-mg and 10-mg warfarin loading doses. *Arch Intern Med* 159: 46–48.

Fennerty A, Campbell IA, Routledge PA (1988). Anticoagulants in venous thromboembolism: Guidelines for optimum treatment. *BMJ* 297: 1285–1288.

National Patient Safety Agency (2008). *Oral anticoagulant therapy patient information booklet*. Available from http://www.nrls .npsa.nhs.uk/resources/?entryid45=61777&q=0%c2%acanti-coagulant%c2%ac (accessed 11 June 2012).

Sweetman S, ed. (2011). *Martindale: the Complete Drug Reference*, 37th edn. Pharmaceutical Press.

Tait RC, Sefcick A (1998). A warfarin induction regimen for out-patient anticoagulation in patients with atrial fibrillation. *Br J Haematol* 101: 450–454.

6

General health advice

Narinder Bhalla

Chapter 6 focuses on providing evidence-based advice to patients on aspects of health, encompassing what the individual can do to ensure that they maintain good health. The scenarios include a range of therapeutic areas and situations that may arise in community pharmacy in particular.

Before you embark on the scenarios below you should read the key references identified. The references will allow you to adequately respond to the issues raised in the OSCE scenarios that follow.

Key references

Healthy lifestyle

The Change4Life website (www.nhs.uk/change4life, accessed 24 May 2012) provides a range of detailed, user friendly information on aspects of good dietary practice designed to help patients lose weight if needed and to eat a healthy diet. Patients who have experienced a cardiovascular event or who are considered to be at risk of such an event, such as those with a high body mass index (BMI) or having other risk factors, may benefit from the advice contained within the site. Pharmacists can act as a point of signposting for individuals seeking advice and support. On a practical level, pharmacists could signpost and then check with the patient how they are using the information to modify their lifestyle and provide additional support and advice as necessary.

Malaria prophylaxis

The NHS Choices weblink (www.nhs.uk/Conditions/Malaria/ Pages/Prevention.aspx, accessed 24 May 2012) provides good background information for patients on symptoms, causes, diagnosis, treatment and prevention of malaria. Community pharmacists are frequently asked to provide advice on prevention of malaria and to advise and provide an appropriate prophylactic drug based upon the level of risk in the area to be visited. For pharmacists the *BNF* provides details on key principles to follow when providing advice about prophylaxis, such as requirements for the area to be visited, and relevant information about the drugs.

Smoking cessation

Pharmacists and students should ensure that as well as reading relevant NICE (National Institute for Health and Clinical Excellence) guidance on smoking cessation services and individual technology appraisals on products, they find out what services are available within the local health economy from primary care, including community pharmacists. As patients often have multiple 'quit attempts', an understanding of the range of options available is valuable in ensuring a pharmacist can provide up-to-date and accurate advice, including signposting to more appropriate services if necessary.

Emergency hormonal contraception

This is a difficult area, with pharmacists having to balance the need to support patients who may be anxious with the need to provide clear, consistent and appropriate advice, taking into account the patient's age, background and possibly cultural and ethnic factors as well as their own beliefs. The following guidance should be read in full before embarking on the OSCE:

- Royal Pharmaceutical Society (2011). *Supply of Levonorgestrel Oral Emergency Contraception as a Pharmacy*

(P) Medicine. Available from http://www.rpharms.com/ home/home.asp (accessed 11 June 2012).

■ General Pharmaceutical Council (2010). *Guidance on the Provision of Pharmacy Services Affected by Religious and Moral Beliefs*. Available from http://www.pharmacyregulation. org/ (accessed 11 June 2012).

■ The NHS Choices Emergency Contraception advice. Available from http://www.nhs.uk/Livewell/Contra ception/Pages/Emergencycontraception.aspx (accessed 24 May 2012).

Managing stress and anxiety (good mental health)

The OSCE scenario focuses on over-the-counter (OTC) treatment options for mental health issues. Pharmacists and students must appreciate that patients considered to have significant mental health issues need immediate referral to their GP. Patients will often ask for particular products they have read about, and it is important that a pharmacist is aware of availability of products and claims of efficacy. The focus should be on evidence-based provision of information. Pharmacists and students should use good-quality evaluated resources to find information (http://www.nhs.uk/livewell/mentalhealth/Pages/Mental healthhome.aspx, accessed 24 May 2012).

Learning Objectives

The following OSCE scenarios assess student consultation, advisory and communication skills. By the end of this chapter you should be able to:

■ provide evidence-based advice to patients presenting in a community pharmacy on a range of areas related to general health advice
■ be aware of appropriate signposting for patients in areas where they may need more specialist or detailed advice

- communicate in clear, professional and empathetic manner, taking into account appropriate patient factors.

For each of the following scenarios, remember to read the scenarios fully and think about the topic before you consider starting your interaction.

Scenario 6.1 Lifestyle advice following a 'heart attack'

Format: Interactive station

Supporting material available to student: *BNF*

Time allowed: 5 minutes

Suggested years of study: undergraduate year 4; pre-registration; postgraduate.

Knowledge and skills tested

- Ability to ask relevant questions
- Knowledge of relevant lifestyle advice
- Ability to give relevant advice
- Communication skills.

Task

You are a community pharmacist working in a local pharmacy. A customer approaches you to ask for lifestyle advice as he has recently experienced a 'heart attack'.

- What questions should you ask before offering advice?
- What lifestyle advice should someone follow after a heart attack?
- What advice would you give to this patient?

Read the notes below after listing the questions you would ask. If you asked the appropriate questions, the patient would have told you that he is a 66-year-old white male. The patient recently had a heart attack (six weeks ago). Current BMI is 27 kg/m².
He takes the following medication supplied by the hospital:

- aspirin 75 mg daily
- ramipril 5 mg daily
- simvastatin 40 mg at night
- bisoprolol 2.5 mg daily
- glyceryl trinitrate sublingual spray 400 micrograms – one or two puffs as required for chest pain.

Other information you may have elucidated about the patient. The patient:

- smokes (20 a day) and has tried to quit several times
- drinks alcohol often (3 beers and a whisky each night)
- knows his diet needs improving
- does not do much exercise
- has a stressful job.

Scenario 6.1 feedback

Questions to be asked/issues clarified before providing advice

- Establish a few basic facts about the individual, including age, ethnic status, weight.
- Establish details of 'heart attack' and medical conditions:
  - When did he experience the 'heart attack'?
  - Are any other medical conditions present (including other cardiovascular conditions such as hypertension)?
  - Are any current regular, as required and OTC medicines taken (including complementary medicines)?

- Establish some lifestyle factors:

  - Daily and weekly alcohol consumption (in units). If the patient is unsure about units then clarify using appropriate verbal or written comparisons
  - Does the patient ever binge drink (clarify definition of binge drinking)?
  - Ask the patient to describe a typical weekly intake of food and drink.
  - Ask about smoking/tobacco consumption status. If the patient is a smoker/tobacco consumer then ask what is smoked/consumed and how often per day. When does the patient have the first smoke/tobacco product of the day?
  - Current weight/BMI is important. Target advice at overweight or obese.
  - Current exercise regimen.

- Establish previous advice:

  - Ask about advice already received from secondary or primary care with regard to healthy lifestyle and patient's level of compliance with such advice. If poor compliance, attempt to establish reasons. By asking these questions you are ensuring the advice can be tailored to the individual's needs.

What lifestyle advice should someone follow after a heart attack?

There are a number of lifestyle changes advised to prevent further problems. Did you cover the following?

Alcohol consumption

- Reduce the amount of alcohol consumed to recommended limits. Men should not regularly drink more than 21 units/week and women should not regularly drink more than 14 units/week.
- Avoid binge drinking, and preferably have a minimum of two alcohol-free days every week.

Diet

- Eat a 'Mediterranean' diet; at least five portions of fruit and vegetables, plenty of nuts, fibre and (oily) fish and limit meat, saturated fat, and salt intake.
- Reduce fat intake (animal fats, fatty foods, e.g. chips, try grilling or baking instead of frying).
- Vitamin supplementation in most people is unnecessary.

Exercise

- Move a little more (i.e. increase the amount of appropriate exercise). Ask the customer whether they have tried to exercise and what they think they can fit into their daily routine.
- Take regular physical activity of moderate intensity for at least 30 minutes per day or 3×10 minutes per day or at least five times a week.
- Maintain body weight within a normal range of BMI $18.5-24.9 \, \text{kg/m}^2$.

Other

- Try to give up smoking. The benefits of stopping smoking are considerable. The patient should be offered the various NHS options on support services to aid their attempt to quit smoking. See also Scenario 6.3.
- Try to reduce stress; suggest stress management techniques.

What advice would you give to this patient?

As this patient has experienced a 'heart attack' recently, it is a good time now to reinforce advice that they will have received. Many NHS secondary care Trusts have cardiac rehabilitation nurses employed to provide advice before discharge and to follow up patients for a while after discharge.

This patient should:

- follow the above advice with regard to losing weight/reducing BMI

- follow the advice with regard to reducing alcohol consumption
- follow the advice with regard to stopping smoking. As he has attempted and failed to quit several times before, a referral to a GP or individual or group service may be appropriate. Options should be discussed with the patient.

Exercise advice is needed but in view of their age and recent 'heart attack' this needs careful evaluation and a principle of starting gently and building up gradually should be followed.

Suggested revision points

- Relevant national advice on good health such as NICE guidance on stopping smoking and the associated technology appraisals for drug treatments.
- Potential benefits of stopping smoking and the likely impact of additional support and drug treatments in order to give properly evaluated advice.
- National websites that patients can be referred to, such as Change4Life (www.nhs.uk/change4life, accessed 6 June 2012). The National Prescribing Centre (http://www.npc.co.uk/, accessed 6 June 2012) also has resources for healthcare professionals to update themselves on the current best advice on lifestyle and the up-to-date evidence base. In addition PRODIGY (http://prodigy.clarity.co.uk/home, accessed 1 October 2012) in the 'Myocardial Infarction – Secondary Prevention' section includes good advice on reducing cardiovascular risk with lifestyle interventions.

Scenario 6.2 Advice on prevention of malaria while abroad

Format: Interactive station

Supporting material available to student: *BNF*

Time allowed: 5 minutes

Suggested years of study: Undergraduate years 3, 4; pre-registration; postgraduate.

Knowledge and skills tested

- Counselling regarding antimalarial dosing
- Non-medical measures of malaria prevention
- Problem-solving.

Task

A customer comes into your pharmacy for some advice about preventing malaria while abroad. They will be travelling to Madagascar in a couple of weeks for a two-week holiday. You discuss with them that they should preferably take Malarone® tablets and other measures used to prevent malaria.

- List the counselling points you would discuss with the customer.
- The customer also asks whether they can take magnesium trisilicate, which they occasionally take for indigestion, with the antimalarials. Address this question.

Scenario 6.2 feedback

Prior to giving advice you should have asked about pre-existing medical conditions and any current medications, to check for any possible problems with malaria prophylaxis. You should have used the *BNF* to locate the advice for malaria prophylaxis. You would have identified that malaria risk is very high for Madagascar, therefore prophylaxis is required.

You should have covered the following counselling points:

- When to start taking the tablets and for how long to continue.
- Malarone® tablets: For an adult or child over 40 kg, start one to two days before entering the area and take during the stay and for one week after returning from the area.

- Dosage: Number of tablets and how many times a day. For adults and children over 40 kg – take one tablet daily.
- Expected side-effects: Abdominal pain, nausea and possibly vomiting or diarrhoea. In addition, cough, headache, dizziness and insomnia.
- Any cautions or precautions (e.g. drug interactions). Diarrhoea or vomiting may result in lack of drug absorption, hence the individual should ensure that they have maximised any non-drug measures.
- Avoid if pregnant or breastfeeding.
- Non-drug measures: Use mosquito nets, advise that long clothing is worn, particularly at dusk and the evening. Consider insect repellents as roll-ons, lotions or sprays containing diethyltoluamide (DEET).

You should also advise that medical advice should be sought if any illness occurs within a year and especially within three months of return from an overseas trip as this could indicate malaria.

When the patient asked for advice regarding the magnesium trisilicate, you should have checked whether there is an interaction. The *BNF* is a suitable place to identify this information. The *BNF* advises that the absorption of proguanil is reduced by oral magnesium salts. Therefore what are the options for you to consider? They include using alternative antacids not containing magnesium, or not taking the Malarone® at the same time of day as the magnesium trisilicate.

Suggested revision points

- *BNF* for general advice and specific drug advice on malaria prophylaxis
- The NHS Choices for good advice that patients can be referred to regarding prophylaxis (http://www.nhs.uk/Conditions/Malaria/Pages/Prevention.aspx, accessed 6 June 2012)
- See PRODIGY online advice on malaria.

Scenario 6.3 Advice on smoking cessation

Format: Interactive station

Supporting material available to student: *BNF* and SPCs for nicotine-replacement products such as gums, lozenges and sprays

Time allowed: 10 minutes

Suggested years of study: Undergraduate year 4; pre-registration; postgraduate.

Knowledge and skills tested

- Knowledge of national guidance related to smoking cessation services
- Knowledge of the specific characteristics of different smoking cessation products to allow appropriate recommendations to be made, taking into account patient factors
- Counselling regarding dose and appropriate use of nicotine-replacement products
- Problem-solving.

Task

You are working as a community pharmacist when you are approached by a customer who wishes to give up smoking to become generally healthier. Using appropriate questions, you are required to gather all relevant information from the customer and offer advice and/or a recommendation.

- What questions do you ask?
- What advice would you give?

Read the notes below after listing the questions you would ask.

- They smoke a few cigarettes a day, mainly socially in the evenings.
- They never smoke before lunch time.
- They do not take any other medicines.
- They have smoked for many years and have tried to give up previously but have not been successful.
- They have tried nicotine gum previously but it gave them a sore throat so they stopped using the gum.
- They would prefer to try something else and their friend has recommended nicotine lozenges.

Scenario 6.3 feedback

What questions do you ask?

- Ask about the number of cigarettes smoked a day (because this influences which formulation you would recommend and the strength of the formulation).
- Ask when the first cigarette of the day is smoked (as this may affect the choice of treatment you recommend) and if the patient wakes up with a craving for a cigarette.
- Check if the patient has any pre-existing medical conditions (patients with diabetes mellitus may need closer monitoring of blood glucose after starting therapy; oral preparations would need to be used with caution in patients with gastrointestinal disorders such as oesophagitis, gastritis, or peptic ulcers as swallowed nicotine may aggravate these conditions).
- Check whether the patient takes any other medication (in case of interactions).
- Ask whether the patient has a preference for the formulation/type of nicotine-replacement product.
- Establish that the sore throat is a possible side-effect of the gum.

What advice would you give?

- Explain to the patient how to use lozenges. They should be sucked until they dissolve, not chewed and not swallowed whole.
- Acidic beverages such as coffee or fruit juice may decrease the absorption of nicotine through the buccal mucosa and should be avoided for 15 minutes before the use of oral nicotine-replacement therapy.
- Common side-effects of lozenges include dizziness and headache, gastrointestinal disturbances (diarrhoea, constipation, indigestion), increased salivation, dry mouth or sore mouth, and less commonly taste disturbance and thirst.
- Signs and symptoms of nicotine withdrawal as they may confuse this with side-effects of the treatment.

Since the patient has already reported sore throat with the gum, he or she may not be keen on the lozenge once made aware that the lozenge can also cause this. As the patient is an infrequent smoker, an alternative immediate-release preparation would be the nasal spray.

Consider also whether it would be appropriate to refer the patient to other smoking cessation services provided locally. You should consider the patient as an individual; such services may be more appropriate for certain patients but not others.

Suggested revision points

- If you do not feel confident in offering advice in this subject area, get to know the nicotine-replacement products available and the differences between them. The *BNF* and the relevant product SPCs give detailed advice.
- NICE Public Health Guidance 10 on Smoking Cessation Services (2008) offers good advice to healthcare workers.

Scenario 6.4 Advice on emergency hormonal contraception

Format: Written station

Supporting material available to student: *BNF*

Time allowed: 10 minutes

Suggested years of study: Pre-registration; postgraduate.

Knowledge and skills tested

- Knowledge of available options for emergency hormonal contraception
- Knowing which patients should be referred for a medical opinion or to other services
- Counselling points.

Task

A customer comes into your pharmacy and asks for advice on the 'morning after pill', which is a service that your pharmacy offers via a Patient Group Direction agreed with the local primary care commission group/GPs.

- What questions would you ask before deciding if emergency hormonal contraception is appropriate?
- If you decide that providing the requested treatment is appropriate, what advice would you offer?
- Which patients should be referred to the GP or other services?

Scenario 6.4 feedback*

Key questions that should be asked

- Who is the levonorgestrel oral emergency contraception for? You can make the supply to someone else (other than

*Royal Pharmaceutical Society guidance is summarised here adapted to this scenario.

the patient directly) if you are satisfied it is a genuine request and the treatment is clinically appropriate for the patient.

- Check the patient's age. If the patient is under 16, she must be referred to a doctor or a family planning clinic to obtain a prescription for emergency contraception or it may be possible to obtain a prescription for emergency contraception unless supply of emergency contraception through the Patient Group Direction is permitted.
- Was unprotected sex/intercourse or failure of a contraceptive method within the last 72 hours? Levonorgestrel oral emergency contraception is most effective if taken within 72 hours of unprotected sex/failure of a contraceptive method (its efficacy decreases with time).
- Is there a possibility that the patient may already be pregnant? Ask the patient if her last period was late, lighter or shorter than usual, or if it was unusual in any way. If there is a possibility that the patient may be pregnant then she should be referred to a doctor or a family planning clinic.
- Has oral emergency contraception been used since the last period? If appropriate, women can take oral emergency contraception more than once within the same menstrual cycle but should be advised about possible cycle disruption.
- Is the patient taking any medicines, including over-the-counter or herbal medicines? The following are examples of drugs that interact with levonorgestrel: carbamazepine, griseofulvin, phenobarbital, phenylbutazone, phenytoin, primidone, rifabutin, rifampicin, ritonavir, St John's wort, ciclosporin. If the patient is taking any of these drugs then she should be referred to a doctor or a family planning clinic.
- Are there any problems that may affect absorption of oral emergency contraception (e.g. vomiting, severe diarrhoea, Crohn's disease)? If yes, then refer to a doctor or a family planning clinic.
- Is there reduced liver function? If yes, then refer to a doctor or a family planning clinic.

- Has there previously been an allergy or other reaction to emergency contraception or levonorgestrel? If yes, then refer to a doctor or a family planning clinic.

What advice would you offer?

- The patient should be advised to take one tablet (1.5 mg), preferably within 12 hours of, and no later than 72 hours following, unprotected intercourse. If vomiting occurs within 2 hours of taking levonorgestrel a replacement dose should be taken.
- You should explain that after taking emergency hormonal contraception:
  - her next period may be late
  - a barrier method of contraception needs to be used until the next period
  - she must see her GP promptly if any lower abdominal pain occurs as this may indicate ectopic pregnancy. She should also see her GP if in the next 3–4 weeks the subsequent menstrual bleed is abnormally light, heavy, brief or absent.

Which patients should be referred?

Patients should be referred to a GP or other family planning services if they:

- are aged under 16 years
- have had unprotected sexual intercourse or experienced failure of a contraceptive method more than 72 hours ago
- are pregnant
- are taking any of the following medicines: carbamazepine, griseofulvin, phenobarbital, phenylbutazone, phenytoin, primidone, rifabutin, rifampicin, ritonavir, St John's Wort, ciclosporin
- have problems that may affect absorption of levonorgestrel oral emergency contraception (e.g. vomiting, severe diarrhoea, Crohn's disease)
- have severe hepatic dysfunction

- have previous allergy or reaction to emergency hormonal contraception or levonorgestrel.

Suggested revision points

- Emergency contraception guidance from NHS Choices
- General Pharmaceutical Council (2010). *Guidance on the Provision of Pharmacy Services Affected by Religious and Moral Beliefs*
- Royal Pharmaceutical Society (2011). *Supply of levonorgestrel oral emergency contraception as a pharmacy (P) medicine.* Available from http://www.rpharms.com/home/home.asp (accessed 11 June 2012).

Scenario 6.5 Managing stress and anxiety (good mental health)

Format: Written station

Supporting material available to student: *BNF*

Time allowed: 10 minutes

Suggested years of study: Pre-registration; postgraduate.

Knowledge and skills tested

- Knowledge of national guidance related to managing depression and generalised anxiety disorder
- Knowledge of the characteristics of St John's wort
- Awareness of the appropriate signposting or referral of patients presenting with mental health conditions.

Task

A 45-year-old man attends your pharmacy wanting some advice on managing stress and asks whether taking 'St John's wort' will help as he has read that this is useful in managing stress and anxiety.

- What questions would you ask of the customer at this point?
- Would you recommend and sell St John's Wort? Give clear reasons for your answer.
- Would you refer the patient to another healthcare professional or service?

Scenario 6.5 feedback

What questions would you ask of the customer at this point?

It is important to establish some basic facts. Relevant questions could include:

- What is your age?
- Are you employed and if so what job do you do?
- Do you have any pre-existing medical conditions?
- Are you on any current medication?
- Have you ever received treatment for anxiety, depression or any other mental health condition?
- What current health or other issue(s) has prompted you to seek advice?

Would you recommend and sell St John's Wort?

St John's Wort *(Hypericum perforatum)* is a herbal remedy on sale to the public and used for the management of anxiety or mild depression. Current NICE guidance on depression (2009) (http://publications.nice.org.uk/depression-in-adults-cg90/guidance, accessed 6 June 2012) states:

> Although there is evidence that St John's Wort may be of benefit in mild or moderate depression, practitioners should:
>
> - not prescribe or advise its use by people with depression because of uncertainty about appropriate doses, persistence of effect, variation in the nature of preparations and

> potential serious interactions with other drugs (including oral contraceptives, anticoagulants and anticonvulsants)
> - advise people with depression of the different potencies of the preparations available and of the potential serious interactions of St John's Wort with other drugs.

In addition, NICE guidance on generalised anxiety disorder does not include St John's Wort within its treatment pathway (http://www.nice.org.uk/nicemedia/live/13314/52599/52599. pdf, accessed 6 June 2012).

Would you refer the patient to another healthcare professional or service?

At this stage the pharmacist should consider whether the patient needs signposting to NHS advice on dealing with stress and anxiety. For example, NHS Choices (http://www. nhs.uk/livewell/mentalhealth/Pages/Mentalhealthhome.aspx, accessed 6 June 2012) offers general advice on dealing with stress and also contains a tool for the patient to assess if they may have depression. A judgement should be made if a referral to the GP is appropriate.

Chapter 6 feedback summary

In Chapter 6 you have attempted scenarios involving:

- healthy lifestyle following a 'heart attack'
- malaria prophylaxis
- smoking cessation
- emergency hormonal contraception
- managing stress and anxiety (good mental health).

You will have learned that knowledge of general aspects of healthy living are important in your role as a pharmacist, and that communicating these aspects effectively to patients is important. People need to be engaged in making lifestyle

Table 6.1   Chapter 6 learning outcomes

Knowledge and skills	More work required	Feel competent
Provide evidence-based advice to patients presenting in a community pharmacy on a range of areas related to general health advice		
Be aware of appropriate signposting for patients in areas where they may need more specialist or detailed advice		
Communicate in clear, professional and empathetic manner taking into account appropriate patient factors		

changes for such changes to be effective. As has been discussed in the introduction and further in Chapters 1 and 2, obtaining a relevant history is very important when offering advice on the issues within this chapter.

Now that you have completed this chapter, assess your competence in the knowledge and skills listed in Table 6.1. Jot down any notes that may help you.

If there are any points that you consider need further work, start a CPD (continuous professional development) cycle now to identify how you can achieve this action.

References and further reading

General Pharmaceutical Council (2010). *Guidance on the Provision of Pharmacy Services Affected by Religious and Moral Beliefs*. Available from http://www.pharmacyregulation.org/ (accessed 11 June 2012).

National Institute for Health and Clinical Excellence guidance on: Public Health Guidance 10 on Smoking Cessation Services

(2008), Depression (2009), Generalised Anxiety Disorder (2011). www.nice.org.uk

NHS. Change4Life. www.nhs.uk/change4life (accessed 24/5/12)

NHS Choices guidance on: *Mental Health*, http://www.nhs .uk/livewell/mentalhealth/Pages/Mentalhealthhome.aspx (accessed 6 June 2012), *Preventing Malaria*, http://www. nhs.uk/Conditions/Malaria/Pages/Prevention.aspx (accessed 24 May 2012), *Emergency Contraception*, http://www.nhs.uk/ Livewell/Contraception/Pages/Emergencycontraception.aspx (accessed 24 May 2012).

Royal Pharmaceutical Society (2011). *Supply of Levonorgestrel Oral Emergency Contraception as a Pharmacy (P) Medicine*. Available from http://www.rpharms.com/home/home.asp (accessed 11 June 2012).

7

Counselling (medication and devices)

Andrzej Kostrzewski

This chapter is focused on scenarios that revolve around the key skills of counselling people about medicines and, where required, demonstrating how to use them. Explanations of using medicines and devices should be brief, but include the essential facts. Instructions should be simple, using illustrations if possible. Pharmacists should support the importance of the medication and the treatment regimen, as well as supporting the patient's motivation to improve his or her health. There can be a number of barriers to this type of communication which need to be kept in mind; for example, hearing what we expect to hear, people interpreting the same instructions in different ways, non-verbal instruction, and physical and emotional barriers.

Every pharmacist has his or her own way of talking to members of the public and you will develop your own way of doing this, or perhaps you have already, but do not worry if this is an area that you find slightly daunting. The more you practise interacting with the public, the easier it will get.

How to approach counselling

- Do not stereotype your patient/carer.
- Find out what the patient knows about the medicine, and what concerns the patient may have. Not all patients need the same information, and some will want to know more detail than others.

- Think about the patient's age and cultural/social background.
- Be clear which medicines are new.
- Be prepared to counsel patients in different contexts (e.g. during a point of sale or point of discharge or after a medicines reconciliation event).
- Use a structured approach.
- Ensure privacy.
- Make sure patients are given the space to ask questions and listen to the patient.

Possible preparation for these stations

You should read the Quick reference guide on *Counselling Patients on Medicines* published by the Royal Pharmaceutical Society (2011) (http://www.rpharms.com/home/home.asp, accessed 11 June 2012).

Take 5 minutes now to consider some of the important factors that you need to consider when counselling members of the public about their medicines.

Before you embark on the following scenarios, look up counselling in some key references.

Key references

Joint Formulary Committee. *British National Formulary*. London: BMJ Group and Pharmaceutical Press.
Summaries of Product Characteristics
Patient Information Leaflets

Learning objectives

The following OSCE scenarios assess a number of skills. By the end of this chapter you should be able to:

- counsel patients about medications
- demonstrate how to use an inhaler, sublingual spray, oral syringe, nasal spray, suppository, eye drops, ear drops
- offer appropriate solutions to everyday questions
- provide written information to support taking medicines.

For each of the following scenarios, remember to read the scenarios fully and think about the topic before you consider starting your interaction.

Scenario 7.1 Inhaler technique

Format: Interactive station

Supporting material available to student: *BNF*, salbutamol metered dose inhaler PIL, prescription stating dosage instructions

Time allowed: 5 minutes

Suggested years of study: Undergraduate years 1–4; pre-registration; postgraduate.

Knowledge and skills tested

- Counselling a customer about a medication
- Describing and demonstrating good inhaler technique.

Task

You have dispensed a salbutamol metered dose inhaler. You need to hand out the inhaler to the customer and counsel them about the medication and on how they should use the inhaler.

Scenario 7.1 feedback

Before you started the interaction, did you read through a Patient Information Leaflet on salbutamol inhaler?

When counselling the customer you should have explained:

- that the salbutamol inhaler is a 'reliever'
- the number of puffs to use during the day, and how often.

You should have also described and demonstrated good inhaler technique. As a minimum you should have offered the following advice:

1. remove the cap
2. shake the inhaler
3. breathe out gently before putting the inhaler in the mouth
4. activate the inhaler as you breathe in
5. continue to inhale after actuation
6. hold breath for as long as is comfortable
7. breathe out slowly
8. repeat the process if a second dose is required.

Have you practised on a placebo metered dose inhaler yourself?

What else would you tell the patient if the inhaler was a corticosteroid?

- Importance of using a 'preventer' inhaler regularly
- How to avoid common side-effects
- Use a spacer to minimise oral thrush
- Rinse mouth with water after inhalation
- Do not interchange brands.

Suggested revision points

- How to use different types of inhalers
- Practise using placebos of different types of inhalers.

Scenario 7.2 Use of a glyceryl trinitrate spray

Format: Interactive station

Supporting material available to student: *BNF*, glyceryl trinitrate spray PIL

Time allowed: 10 minutes

Suggested years of study: Undergraduate years 2–4; pre-registration; postgraduate.

Knowledge and skills tested

- How to use a glyceryl trinitrate spray
- Storage and side-effects of glyceryl trinitrate spray.

Task

You are running a session on cardiac medicines for the cardiac rehabilitation group at your hospital. You are required to explain what a glyceryl trinitrate (GTN) sublingual spray is used for, and to show the participants how to use it. You are also asked about side-effects and storage of the medicine.

Scenario 7.2 feedback

You should have advised the patients that GTN spray is used to prevent and relieve chest pain or angina. You should have explained how it works in plain English terms. Appropriate language might include: it 'opens' up the blood vessels so that the heart is under less strain.

- In terms of dosage, did you give advice on:

  - when to use the spray (e.g. when required to relieve chest pain, which may be at the onset of an attack, or prior to an event known to precipitate chest pain)
  - the number of sprays to use at a time, and on the time interval between doses
  - repeating the dose, and on action to take if repeated doses do not relieve the pain?

- When demonstrating the use of the spray did you:

  - remove the cap and hold the spray upright
  - explain there is no need to shake the canister
  - advise patients to prime the spray before using for the first time
  - advise patients to spray one spray under the tongue and close the mouth

- advise the patients to sit down and rest until the pain subsides?

■ How did you advise the patients to store the medicine?

- Do not store above 25°C, do not freeze
- Do not attempt to puncture the canister
- Do not use after the expiry date.

■ Did you suggest they should carry the spray with them at all times?

■ Did you advise patients to obtain a further supply before the old one runs out?

You should have advised the patient that the most common side-effects of the spray are throbbing headache, flushing and dizziness. It would be appropriate to add that people tend to get used to the headache, or that it becomes less severe with use of the spray.

Suggested revision points

■ How to use glyceryl trinitrate sprays
■ Practise using a placebo.

Scenario 7.3 Using an oral syringe

Format: Interactive station

Supporting material available to student: *BNF*, oral syringe instruction sheet

Time allowed: 5 minutes

Suggested years of study: Undergraduate years 1–4; pre-registration; postgraduate.

Knowledge and skills tested

■ Correctly issue a dispensed item to a customer
■ Ability to counsel a customer about a medication

- Ability to explain/demonstrate how to use the oral syringe device.

Task

You have prepared a prescription for Augmentin® 125/31 SF suspension for a male child (2 mL t.d.s. for 5 days). The prescription is valid, and the dose is correct for the child's age and weight. It is being used to treat respiratory tract infection. His parent has arrived to collect the prescription. You need to hand out the prescription to the parent and counsel them on how they should use the oral syringe.

Scenario 7.3 feedback

- Did you check whether the child is allergic to penicillin?
- Did you inform the parent that:
  - the medicine is an antibiotic (penicillin-type)
  - the medicine should be used for 5 days (complete the course)
  - the dose is 2 mL three times a day, given using an oral syringe
  - the medicine should be stored in the fridge.

It may be tempting in scenarios such as these to launch into how to use the oral syringe, forgetting the essential information of what the medicine is, the dose to take, and any other advice.

Did you cover the following points regarding using the oral syringe?

1. Shake the bottle, remove bottle cap, insert the bung (bottle adapter) firmly into the bottle neck.
2. Take the syringe and pull back the plunger a little way. Push the oral syringe into the hole in the bung, and turn the bottle upside down with syringe in place.
3. To draw the medicine into the syringe, pull the plunger back beyond the point on the scale that corresponds to the dose prescribed for the child.

4. Then remove air bubbles/push back to the required point on the scale (top of black ring lines up with dose required).
5. Turn the bottle back the right way up and withdraw the syringe from the bung, holding the syringe by the barrel rather than by the plunger.
6. With child upright, gently put the tip of the syringe into the child's mouth, to the inside of the child's cheek.
7. Slowly and gently push the plunger down to gently squirt the medicine into the inside of the child's cheek. Allow them to swallow it (bit by bit).
8. Do not squirt it to the back of the neck of throat in case the child chokes.
9. Remove the syringe from the child's mouth.
10. Remove the bung from the bottle.
11. Wash the oral syringe and bung in warm water and allow to dry.

Suggested revision points

■ Counselling patients and carers about use of antibiotics
■ Use of oral syringes. If you are not familiar with demonstrating the use of oral syringes see the leaflets produced by manufacturers of the devices.

Scenario 7.4 Nasal spray

Format: Interactive station

Supporting material available to student: *BNF*, product information leaflet

Time allowed: 5 minutes

Suggested years of study: Undergraduate years 1–4; pre-registration; postgraduate.

Knowledge and skills tested

■ Use of corticosteroids in the management of hayfever
■ How to use nasal sprays.

Task

A customer arrives to collect a prescription for a Rhinocort Aqua® nasal spray. The dose is two sprays into each nostril once daily. The customer has hayfever, for which they occasionally take the antihistamine loratadine. They have never used a nasal spray before.

What would you tell the patient about the medication and how would you counsel the patient on how to use the device?

Scenario 7.4 feedback

You should have:

- stated the name of spray and what it is (corticosteroid)
- given dosage instructions
- explained how it works nasally (reduces inflammation/congestion)
- explained that it is best used preventively and may take a few days to work
- demonstrated how to use the spray.

Did you find instructions on how to use the device in the Patient Information Leaflet?

How to use the spray

Priming the nozzle. Before using for the first time:

1. Shake the bottle and remove the protective cap.
2. Hold the bottle upright.
3. Pump the nozzle up and down 5–10 times, spraying into the air until you see an even mist.

The priming effect remains for about 24 hours. Leaving a longer gap before the next dose will require you to prime the nozzle again. This time spray into air just once.

Using Rhinocort Aqua®

1. Put the tip of the nozzle into the nostril. Spray once. Use the spray in other nostril the same way. You do not need to breathe in at the same time as you spray.
2. Wipe nozzle with a clean tissue and replace cap.
3. Store bottle in upright position.

Suggested revision points

■ Counselling patient about use of nasal sprays.

Scenario 7.5 Using a suppository

Format: Interactive station

Supporting material available to student: *BNF*, PIL for diclofenac suppositories

Time allowed: 5 minutes

Suggested years of study: Undergraduate years 2–4; pre-registration; postgraduate.

Knowledge and skills tested

■ Counselling how to administer suppositories
■ Communicating sensitive issues.

Task

You have dispensed a prescription for diclofenac 100 mg suppositories for an adult patient. When handing the prescription in, the patient told you that they have not used this type of medication before and would like you to explain how it is used. Using the Patient Information Leaflet provided, you need to counsel the patient on how to administer the diclofenac suppositories.

Scenario 7.5 feedback

Imagine you are in this situation and write down below the points you would cover. Did you include the following points?

1. Go to the toilet and empty your bowels if necessary.
2. Wash your hands.
3. Remove any foil or plastic wrapping from the suppository.
4. Either squat or lie on your side with one leg bent and the other straight.
5. Gently but firmly push the suppository into the rectum, pointed end first.
6. Push it in far enough so that it does not slip out.
7. Close your legs and sit or lie still for a few minutes.
8. If you feel your body wanting to expel the suppository, lie still and press your buttocks together.
9. Wash your hands again.
10. Try not to empty your bowels for at least an hour.

Suggested revision points

■ Counselling patients about inserting a suppository. Consider the language you use because some patients find this type of administration difficult or embarrassing.

Scenario 7.6 Using eye drops

Format: Interactive station

Supporting material available to student: *BNF*, PIL for Cosopt®

Time allowed: 5 minutes

Suggested years of study: Undergraduate years 1–4; pre-registration; postgraduate.

Knowledge and skills tested

- Counselling and advice regarding eye drops
- Demonstrate how to use eye drops.

Task

You have prepared a prescription for Cosopt® eye drops for Mr A (1 drop both eyes b.d.). It is being used to treat glaucoma. Someone has approached the counter to collect the prescription. You need to hand out the eye drops to the customer and counsel them on how they should use the eye drops.

Imagine you are having a conversation with the person who has come to collect the prescription.

- How would you start the conversation?
- What would you tell the patient about the medication?

If the customer had been asked the relevant questions they would have told you that they:

- are the patient
- are not asthmatic
- do not take any regular medication
- are allergic to penicillin
- have not used eye drops before
- do not wear soft contact lenses.

Scenario 7.6 feedback

When handing over a prescription you should always confirm the patient's name and address.

You should have asked or advised:

- who the prescription is for
- what the eye drops are for. How do you explain in lay language what glaucoma is? You could say something like

'glaucoma is a condition where the pressure in the eye is raised'.

- how to use the eye drops (one drop twice a day into each eye).
- about any allergies or contra-indications, e.g. asthma.
- about side-effects (e.g. eye stinging, burning, unusual taste, pain, itching, irritation, dry or red eyes).

Regarding use of the eye drops, did you advise that patients should:

1. Wash hands before using eye drops; tilt head back and look upwards, pull down lower lid to create a pocket.
2. Hold bottle above eye (do not let it touch the eye), squeeze one drop into the pocket.
3. Dispose of the eye drops after 28 days.

Suggested revision points

- The different types of glaucoma
- How to instil eye drops
- How medicines lower raised pressure in the eye
- Review any drug interactions with oral medicines.

Scenario 7.7 Ear drops

Format: Written or interactive station

Supporting material available to student: *BNF*

Time allowed: 5 minutes

Suggested years of study: Undergraduate years 2–4; pre-registration; postgraduate.

Knowledge and skills tested

- Counselling a parent and child
- Counselling patients to use ear drops.

Task

You are about to hand out a prescription to a customer who is the parent of an 8-year-old boy. You need to counsel the parent and child about the medicine. The child has otitis externa, which is not infected.

The prescription is for: Betnesol® ear drops, 3 drops left ear every 3 hours for 5 days (1 OP).

You are also asked by the parent whether they need to set the alarm clock throughout the night to use the drops during sleep time.

Scenario 7.7 feedback

You should have explained:

- this is an anti-inflammatory medication, called Betnesol®
- the dose is 3 drops into the left ear every 3 hours for 5 days.
- how to use:

    - the ear drops should be at body temperature (37°C)
    - tilt head to one side or lie on a bed with affected ear towards the ceiling
    - with one hand pull the top of the ear upwards and outwards to straighten the ear canal
    - place drops in the ear canal (squeeze bottle very gently if necessary)
    - keep head tilted for a minute or two to let drops be absorbed
    - do not put cotton wool into the entrance of the ear canal

- discard 4 weeks after opening (i.e. if problem recurs do not use same bottle).

How did you respond to the question about waking to use the drops? Did you advise to use only during waking hours? This reflects the pragmatic approach used in practice.

Did you use appropriate language?

Did you give all the essential information, clearly and inspiring confidence?

See the list of how to approach counselling at the start of this chapter.

Suggested revision points

- Aetiology and pathophysiology of otitis externa
- How to explain the use of a medicine to a child.

Scenario 7.8 Alendronate

Format: Interactive station

Supporting material available to student: *BNF*

Time allowed: 5 minutes

Suggested years of study: Undergraduate years 2–4; pre-registration; postgraduate.

Knowledge and skills tested

- Explanation of a disease and mechanism of action of a medicine in lay terms
- Ability to counsel a patient about a medication and possible side-effects.

Task

Mrs Smith, a 70-year-old patient whom you have not seen for several weeks, presents a new prescription for alendronate 70 mg tablets. She explains that she has been in hospital with a fractured neck of femur, and that a diagnosis of osteoporosis has been made. She has not had alendronate tablets before and says she does not understand how the medication can help. You are required to:

- Explain to the patient the reason for using alendronate in osteoporosis

- Counsel the patient about how to take the medication, and possible side-effects.

Scenario 7.8 feedback

Did you:

- explain that alendronate is used for the treatment of osteoporosis (it works by strengthening bone therefore helping to prevent fractures)
- explain that it is taken once weekly on the same day each week
- emphasise that it must be taken first thing in the morning 30 minutes before any food or other medication, with a full glass of water
- advise the patient to sit or stand upright for 30 minutes after taking
- advise the patient that it is a long-term treatment and may be continued for several years
- advise the patient about the risk of oesophageal ulceration and to seek help if symptoms of this occur
- advise the patient that bone, muscle and/or joint pain is very common?

Suggested revision points

- What is osteoporosis?
- Non-pharmacological treatment of osteoporosis
- Possible drug interactions with alendronate
- How to administer calcium supplements with alendronate
- Review the counselling advice given in the *BNF* for bisphosphonates.

Scenario 7.9 Warfarin

Format: Interactive station

Supporting material available to student: *BNF*, oral anti-coagulant therapy patient information booklet

Time allowed: 10 minutes

Suggested years of study: Undergraduate years 2–4; pre-registration; postgraduate.

Knowledge and skills tested

- Counselling patients about warfarin
- Use of the yellow anticoagulant therapy book.

Task

A patient presents to your community pharmacy having been started on warfarin for deep vein thrombosis in hospital a week earlier. They may have been given 1 mg tablets of warfarin which are labelled 'take as directed'. The patient shows you the book which indicates a dosage of 3 mg daily.

The patient asks you to repeat advice on how to take the medicine, and asks why the treatment is needed and also why blood tests are needed. Address these questions and take the opportunity to go through the information in the yellow book with the patient.

Imagine you are having this interaction and write down what you tell the patient before reading the feedback.

Scenario 7.9 feedback

Did you cover the following?

- How to take warfarin:

    - correct dose and frequency
    - the time of day to take warfarin
    - what to do if a dose is missed.

- Going through the contents of the *Oral Anticoagulant Therapy Patient Information Booklet?* Key points include: emergency advice, condition, medicine description, how anticoagulant is monitored, target INR, serious side-effects, things that can affect the control of anticoagulation.

■ The reason for taking warfarin, explained in lay language.
■ Why are blood tests needed?

  – Starting to take a medicine known as an anticoagulant
  – Anticoagulants prevent harmful blood clots occurring by making the blood take longer to clot
  – The test that measure how quickly the blood clots is called the INR
  – INR means international normalised ratio
  – The dose of the anticoagulant depends on your INR test result.

Suggested revision points

■ Treatment of deep vein thrombosis
■ *Oral Anticoagulant Therapy Patient Information Booklet*, available from the National Patient Safety Agency website (see References).

Scenario 7.10 Prednisolone reducing dose

Format: Interactive station

Supporting material available to student: e.g. *BNF*

Time allowed: 5 minutes

Suggested years of study: Undergraduate years 2–4; pre-registration; postgraduate.

Knowledge and skills tested

■ Communication skills
■ Counselling patients about how to take medicines.

Task

A customer has come to collect a prescription for:

- Asacol® MR 400 mg t.d.s. (84)
- Prednisolone 5 mg tab. 25 mg o.d. for 5 days, reducing by 5 mg every 3 days then stop.

You need to counsel the customer about the dispensed medication. The patient also asks you why they have to reduce the dose of prednisolone gradually, why can't they 'just stop them like any other tablets'?

Scenario 7.10 feedback

In your medication counselling did you cover the following?

- Explain the names and doses of both drugs
- Give advice regarding reporting any symptoms of blood disorders when taking mesalazine (Asacol® MR) (e.g. unexplained bleeding, bruising, purpura, sore throat, fever or malaise)
- Explain the reducing dose of prednisolone clearly
- Advise the patient that prednisolone is best taken in the morning
- The contents of a Steroid Treatment Card (see *BNF*)
- Mood and behaviour changes.

Did you answer the question appropriately in language suitable for the patient (to reduce the risk of adrenal suppression, or similar words, e.g. to allow time for body to recover, to prevent 'shock')?

Suggested revision points

- The physiology of adrenal suppression
- Main side-effects of glucocorticoids

- The different preparations of mesalazine available
- Steroid Treatment Cards – use and content.

Scenario 7.11 Medicines adherence chart

Format: Written station

Supporting material available to student: e.g. *BNF*

Time allowed: 5 minutes

Suggested years of study: Undergraduate years 2–4; pre-registration; postgraduate.

Knowledge and skills tested

- Explaining what medicines are for in lay terms
- Transcribing data from a prescription on to a compliance chart accurately
- Identification of relevant information to give patients.

Task

Mrs Smith is being discharged from hospital following admission for an acute exacerbation of asthma. You are counselling her about the medicines she needs to take on leaving hospital (as listed on the prescription). Mrs Smith asks you to fill in a chart to explain what the medicines are for and how to take them. You should fill in the chart (Table 7.1) provided with the relevant information you wish to give Mrs Smith.

The medicines listed on the prescription are:

- Terbutaline turbohaler 500 mcg q.d.s.
- Budesonide turbohaler 400 mcg b.d.

Table 7.1 Medicines adherence chart for Scenario 7.11

Medicine	What it's for/ how it works	How much to take/use and when			
		Morning	Midday	Afternoon	Evening	Comments/ other information

Table adapted from Department of Health (2005). *Medicines Use Review: Understand your medicines.* Available from: www.dh.gov.uk/prod_consum_dh/groups/dh_digitalassets/@dh/@en/documents/digitalasset/dh_412844.pdf (accessed 11 June 2012).

Scenario 7.11 feedback

Did you complete the chart as shown in Table 7.2?

Additional information to be given to the patient before discharge would include:

- You should never let your medications run out.
- Relievers rescue you from breathing problems, they do not reduce inflammation.
- Preventers only work if they are taken every day, they will not provide instant relief but work continuously to help your symptoms.

Suggested revision points

- How to use a turbohaler
- Explain the difference between reliever and preventer inhalers.

Chapter 7 feedback summary

In Chapter 7 you have looked at counselling patients about their medication and devices. You will have learned that counselling effectively takes practice. Even apparently simple prescriptions can require a lot of advice and support. Patient Information Leaflets are useful supporting information when counselling, and can be recommended to patients for further reading at home. Medicines come in many different formulations and presentations, and pharmacists need to know their products well in order to communicate key information to patients and/or carers.

Now that you have completed this chapter, assess your competence in the knowledge and skills listed in Table 7.3. Jot down any notes that may help you.

If there are any points that you consider need further work, start a CPD (continuous professional development) cycle now to identify how you can achieve this action.

Table 7.2 Example completed chart for Scenario 7.11

| Medicine | What it's for/ how it works | How much to take/use and when | | | | Comments/ other information |
		Morning	Midday	Afternoon	Evening	
Terbutaline turbohaler 500 mcg per inhalation (puff)	To open up/ relax the airways, making breathing easier (reliever)	One dose (inhalation)	One dose (inhalation)	One dose (inhalation)	One dose (inhalation)	The powder in turbohalers is very fine so you might find that you do not taste anything after using the inhaler. Hold the turbohaler upright to load it with the medicine. The reliever works quickly but the effect lasts only a few hours
Budesonide turbohaler 400 mcg per inhalation (puff)	A corticosteroid to reduce inflammation in the lungs; used to prevent symptoms (preventer)	One dose (inhalation)			One dose (inhalation)	Rinse mouth after use to reduce the risk of oral thrush. Use regularly and do not stop without your doctor's advice, even if the asthma is better

Table 7.3 Chapter 7 learning outcomes

Knowledge and skills	More work required	Feel competent
Counsel patients about medications		
Demonstrate how to use an inhaler, sublingual spray, oral syringe, nasal spray, eye drops, ear drops, and a suppository.		
Offer appropriate solutions to everyday questions		
Provide written information to support taking medicines		

References and further reading

Baxa Ltd. (2007) *Exacta-Med® Oral/Enteral Dispensers*. Available from: http://www.baxa.com/betterusebaxa/downloads/Oral%20Enteral%20IFU%202007.pdf (accessed 3 June 2012).

Department of Health (2005). *Medicines Use Review: Understand your medicines*. Available from: www.dh.gov.uk/prod_consum_dh/groups/dh_digitalassets/@dh/@en/documents/digitalasset/dh_4126844.pdf (accessed 11 June 2012).

Keeling D, Baglin T, Tait C *et al.* (2011). Guidelines on oral anticoagulation with warfarin – fourth edition. *British Journal of Haematology*. doi:10.1111/j.1365–2141.2011.08753.x. Available from: http://www.bcshguidelines.com/documents/warfarin_4th_ed.pdf (accessed 12 June 2012).

National Institute for Health and Clinical Excellence (2009). *Medicines Adherence: Involving patients in decisions about prescribed medicines and supporting adherence*. Clinical Guideline 76. Available from: http://www.nice.org.uk/nicemedia/live/11766/43042/43042.pdf (accessed 12 June 2012).

National Patient Safety Agency (2008). *Oral Anticoagulant Therapy Patient Information Booklet.* Available from: http://www .nrls.npsa.nhs.uk/resources/?entryid45=61777&q=0%c2% acanticoagulant%c2%ac (accessed 11 June 2012).

National Pharmacy Association (2006). *Supporting Self Care: Helping people to help themselves and responding to symptoms in the pharmacy.* London: NPA.

Royal Pharmaceutical Society (2011). *Counselling Patients on Medicines. A quick reference guide.* Available from: http://www .rpharms.com/home/home.asp (accessed 11 June 2012).

8

Problems involving calculations

Nina Walker and Jenny Silverthorne

Chapter 8 is focused on scenarios that require you to use numeracy skills. Numeracy is a crucial skill for a pharmacist and you need to be confident in how you tackle problems where calculations are involved. As with most things, the more you practise the easier it gets.

Take 5 minutes now to consider how confident you are with calculations. Is it an area that you find very easy or is it something that you really need to work at? Remember that even if you use a calculator in your practice usually it is worth while getting into the habit of doing a mental check so that you know roughly what answer you are aiming for. Now consider some of the situations where you have recently come across calculations and think about what aspects in particular you find challenging. Remember that the use of calculators in OSCEs may not be permitted (check local arrangements).

Before you embark on the following scenarios, make sure you are familiar with some key references. Remember, some of these references are available online.

Key references

Joint Formulary Committee. *British National Formulary*. London: BMJ Group and Pharmaceutical Press.
Summaries of Product Characteristics (SPC).

Learning objectives

The following OSCE scenarios assess your problem-solving skills in relation to problems involving calculations. By the end of this chapter you should be able to:

- extract key data in order to correctly solve a calculation problem
- use formulae to manipulate data presented in a pharmacy situation
- identify appropriate reference sources to use in different situations
- retrieve information efficiently and explain this information effectively.

For each of the following scenarios, remember to read the scenarios fully and think about the topic before you consider starting your interaction.

Scenario 8.1 Iron-deficiency anaemia

Format: Written station

Supporting material available to student: *BNF*

Time allowed: 5 minutes

Suggested years of study: Undergraduate years 1–2.

Knowledge and skills tested

- Treatment of iron-deficiency anaemia
- Ability to make recommendations regarding management of a patient with swallowing difficulties.

Task

While working as a ward pharmacist you are approached by a junior doctor who asks for advice regarding initiating iron therapy. The patient is 32-year-old Mr J, who has newly diagnosed iron-deficiency anaemia.

Answer the following questions:

1. What is the *BNF* recommended treatment for iron deficiency anaemia expressed as elemental iron?
2. How does the *BNF* suggest this is customarily given? Give a dose and frequency for administration.
3. The patient is unable to swallow tablets and the doctor wants to prescribe a liquid preparation. Give a recommendation including product and dose.
4. For how long should treatment be continued?
5. What counselling would you want to give to Mr J about the preparation you have recommended?

Scenario 8.1 feedback

1. What is the BNF recommended treatment for iron deficiency anaemia expressed as elemental iron?

You should use the *BNF* to find that the recommended treatment is 100–200 mg of elemental iron daily.

2. How does the BNF suggest this is customarily given? Give a dose and frequency for administration

This is customarily given as dried ferrous sulphate 200 mg (=65 mg elemental iron) three times daily.

3. The patient is unable to swallow tablets and the doctor wants to prescribe a liquid preparation. Give a recommendation including product and dose

Any of the following would be suitable (products, dosage):

■ Fersamal® Syrup, 10 mL twice daily
■ Galfer® Syrup, 10 mL one to two times daily
■ Sytron® Elixir, 5 mL increasing gradually to 10 mL three times daily

Ironorm® drops would not be appropriate as the 0.6 mL dose gives only 15 mg elemental iron per day and is for prophylactic use and Niferex® Elixir is not suitable because it is not available on the NHS.

4. For how long should treatment be continued?

Treatment should be continued until the patient's haemoglobin returns to the normal range, and then for a further three months to replenish the iron stores within the body.

5. What counselling would you want to give to Mr J about the preparation you have recommended?

Mr J should be told:

- the dose and frequency of his medication
- when to take the medication (time of day and in relation to food)
- that iron preparations can cause an upset stomach – constipation or diarrhoea may occur
- that iron salts cause blackening of the stools
- that some medications, such as indigestion remedies, interact with iron preparations.

Suggested revision points

- Retrieval of information regarding different preparations from various sources
- Management of different anaemias
- The difference between prophylaxis and treatment of anaemia
- Identification of symbols used in the *BNF*, such as that used for products that cannot be prescribed on the NHS.

Scenario 8.2 Benzodiazepine withdrawal

Format: Written station

Supporting material available to student: *BNF*

Time allowed: 5 minutes

Suggested years of study: Undergraduate year 4; pre-registration; postgraduate.

Knowledge and skills tested

- Withdrawal of benzodiazepine therapy
- Numeracy.

Task

You are a pharmacist in a mental health unit. A patient is admitted who has been prescribed oxazepam 15 mg t.d.s. for 11 months. You are asked to devise a programme for withdrawing this medicine.

- Outline the steps involved in withdrawal
- Identify two symptoms that should be monitored during withdrawal.

Scenario 8.2 feedback

You should have identified the need to convert oxazepam to diazepam. Information on equivalent dosages of benzodiazepines is given in the *BNF*.

The *BNF* states the approximate equivalent dose of oxazepam 15 mg is diazepam 5 mg. Therefore, for this patient an approximate equivalent dose of diazepam would be 15 mg, preferably at night. You should also advise dosage reduction at intervals of 2–3 weeks, in steps of about one eighth (range of one tenth to one quarter) of the daily dose.

Symptoms that could be monitored during withdrawal include: insomnia, loss of appetite, anxiety, tremor, perspiration, tinnitus, perceptual disturbances. It would also be appropriate to mention benzodiazepine withdrawal syndrome.

Suggested revision points

- How to locate dosage conversion tables in the *BNF*, for example for opioids (e.g. oral morphine to subcutaneous diamorphine or transdermal fentanyl); oral theophylline to intravenous aminophylline; dexamethasone to prednisolone

■ Familiarity with location of appropriate of information according to *BNF* index

■ Benzodiazepines indications

■ Characteristics of benzodiazepine withdrawal syndrome.

Scenario 8.3 Tuberculosis treatment dosages

Format: Written station

Supporting material available to student: *BNF*

Time allowed: 5 minutes

Suggested years of study: Undergraduate years 2–4; pre-registration; postgraduate.

Knowledge and skills tested

■ Numeracy (checking doses of prescribed medications)

■ Data retrieval and interpretation from the *BNF*.

Task

You are presented with an FP10 prescription for a child. You need to check whether the doses of tuberculosis (TB) medication for the four-month continuation phase are appropriate for the patient. They are on an unsupervised regimen.

The details on the prescription are as follows:

Title, Forename, Surname and Address: Mr Daniel Potter, 12 The Avenue, Anytown, AN5 4DF
Age: 5 years
Medication details: Supply 4/12; isoniazid 300 mg o.d.; supply 4/12 rifampicin 180 mg o.d.

The necessary prescriber's details are present and correct, and the prescription is signed and in date. The infection is classed as fully sensitive, however a combination product is not appropriate for this patient.

You are required to answer the following questions:

1. What is the weight of an average child of this age?
2. Calculate the isoniazid dose. Is the prescribed dose appropriate? Explain.
3. Calculate the rifampicin dose. Is the prescribed dose appropriate? Explain.

Scenario 8.3 feedback

TB treatment doses are dependent on two key factors:

- Initial vs. continuation phase.

    - Look now to see which antibiotics are typically used in the initial phase and in the continuation phase.
    - What is the duration of treatment for each phase?

- Supervised vs. unsupervised treatment. There are two types of regimen depending on how much supervision is needed. Refer to the *BNF* for information on supervision.

1. What is the weight of an average child of this age?

Where do you find this information?

The answer is 18 kg, which can be found in the table at the back of the *BNF* listed under 'prescribing for children'.

2. Calculate the isoniazid dose. Is the prescribed dose appropriate? Explain

The recommended dose is 10 mg/kg daily (max 300 mg/day). For an 18 kg child the dose is 180 mg daily. The prescribed dosage of 300 mg o.d. is too high.

3. Calculate the rifampicin dose. Is the prescribed dose appropriate? Explain

The recommended dose is 10 mg/kg daily (max 450 mg/day if bodyweight under 50 kg). At 18 kg the dose is 180 mg/day. The prescribed dosage is correct for the weight of the child.

Suggested revision points

- How to locate key dosage information in the notes section of the *BNF*
- Dosage calculations for supervised and unsupervised tuberculosis treatment regimens.

Scenario 8.4 Antibiotic displacement values

Format: Written station

Supporting material available to student: SPC for cefotaxime, calculator

Time allowed: 5 minutes

Suggested years of study: Undergraduate year 4; pre-registration; postgraduate.

Knowledge and skills tested

- Data retrieval and interpretation from a SPC
- Numeracy (dosage calculations).

Task

A junior doctor approaches you (the pharmacist) to ask for advice on dosing and preparation of cefotaxime injection. He needs to prescribe cefotaxime injection for a child with a chest infection. The child's weight is 15 kg and he is 3 years old. The doctor wishes to administer intravenous (IV) bolus injections. The child has no known allergies, and no renal impairment.

Using the SPC for cefotaxime, answer the following questions.

1. What dose and frequency of administration is specified in the SPC for a child of this age in view of the infection indicated?

2. In order to administer the dose the doctor has a 1 g vial

    (a) What diluent should be used to reconstitute the injection?
    (b) What volume of diluent should be added?
    (c) What is the displacement volume when preparing the 1 g injection?
    (d) What is the final available volume once the 1 g vial is reconstituted?

3. If the doctor wanted to administer a dose of 750 mg as an initial IV bolus to this child, what volume of cefotaxime injection would be administered assuming a 1 g vial is used?

Scenario 8.4 feedback

1. What dose and frequency of administration is specified in the SPC for a child of this age in view of the infection indicated?

For children the SPC advises 100–150 mg/kg per day in 2–4 divided doses. In very severe infection doses of up to 200 mg/kg per day may be required.

Where did you find this information? This can usually be found in section 4.2 of the SPC 'Posology and method of administration'.

2. In order to administer the dose the doctor has a 1 g vial:

a. What diluent should be used to reconstitute the injection?
Water for Injections

b. What volume of diluent should be added?   4 mL.

c. What is the displacement volume when preparing the 1 g injection?   0.5 mL.

d. What is the final available volume once the 1 g vial is reconstituted?   4.5 mL.

3. If the doctor wanted to administer a dose of 750 mg as an initial IV bolus to this child what volume of cefotaxime injection would be administered assuming a 1 g vial is used

One gram of the reconstituted vial contains 4.5 mL of solution; 1000 mg in 4.5 mL; therefore 750 mg in 3.4 mL of solution (rounded up from 3.375 mL).

Suggested revision points

- Navigation of SPCs, finding key information
- Definition of displacement volume.

Scenario 8.5 Changing formulations (epilepsy)

Format: Interactive station

Supporting material available to student: *BNF*

Time allowed: 5 minutes

Suggested years of study: Undergraduate years 1–4; pre-registration; postgraduate.

Knowledge and skills tested

- Data retrieval and interpretation from the *BNF*
- Numeracy (calculation of the correct dose conversions).

Task

You are working in a community pharmacy when a patient approaches you with a query about a change in their medication.

The patient has epilepsy, for which they take Tegretol® 300 mg b.d. The patient has just visited their GP because of a sickness 'bug' which has meant that they have not been able to 'keep the Tegretol® tablets down'. The GP has prescribed

Tegretol® suppositories 375 mg b.d. for a few days to be used instead of the tablets. The patient does not understand why the dose of the suppositories is different from that of the tablets. You are asked to explain this apparent change in dosage.

What, if any, further questions would you ask the patient? (Read the information below after you have considered other questions you would ask.)

If you asked appropriate questions the patient may tell you that she or he:

■ has taken Tegretol® for epilepsy for about 5 years

■ has well-controlled epilepsy

■ has not had any therapeutic drug monitoring done for years

■ has used suppositories before so knows how to use them

■ has not take any other medicines and does not have any other medical conditions.

Scenario 8.5 feedback

Considering each question in turn. The patient has been taking Tegretol® for 5 years, and is thus likely to be stabilised on the treatment. Their epilepsy is well controlled and you would not expect a dose change. As the patient is not taking any other medicines, it is unlikely that any interactions can account for the dose change.

■ Did you locate the relevant section in the *BNF*? You should be looking for information on the equivalence of a Tegretol® suppository to a tablet. Each 125 mg suppository is approximately equivalent to a 100 mg tablet. Therefore, a 375 mg dose by suppository is approximately equivalent to a 300 mg dose using tablets.

■ How did you explain the equivalence? What words did you use? Suitable explanations might include phrases such as 'They will give the same effect' or 'same level of control'.

- Did you consider whether there are any implications for the effectiveness of the medication?
- Did you advise on any monitoring requirements? Although the equivalence calculated should provide the required dosage, clinical response should also be noted and final dosage adjustments made accordingly.

Suggested revision points

- Medicines for which the dosage given is different with different formulations (e.g. phenytoin liquid/capsules, citalopram tablets/drops, beclometasone metered dose inhaler – CFC-containing/CFC-free).
- Counselling techniques for explaining concepts such as equivalence to patients.

Scenario 8.6 Antibiotic dosage in renal impairment

Format: Written or interactive station

Supporting material available to student: SPC for ceftazidime, calculator

Time allowed: 5 minutes

Suggested years of study: Undergraduate years 3–4; pre-registration; postgraduate.

Knowledge and skills tested

- Data retrieval and interpretation
- Numeracy.

Task

You are asked by a junior doctor on a ward visit to advise on the dose of intravenous ceftazidime for a male patient. The registrar has recommended 1 g t.d.s. for a respiratory tract infection, but the patient has some degree of renal impairment.

The patient's serum creatinine has been 150 micromol/L for the past 3 days. Weight 62 kg, age 62 years. He is not obese and has no other notable clinical conditions. He is not neutropenic. You need to address the questions using the equations provided.

1. Calculate the creatinine clearance using the equation provided. Renal function can be estimated using the Cockroft–Gault equation:

Creatinine clearance (mL/min) = F × ([140 − age (years)] × weight [kg]) ÷ serum creatinine (micromol/L)

where $F = 1.04$ in females, and 1.23 in males.

2. Use the SPC to recommend an appropriate dose.
3. Explain how you reached your decision in question 2.

Scenario 8.6 feedback

Using the equation given, the creatinine clearance is 39.6552 mL/min. Beware of any corrections required (e.g. to one or two decimal places).

The SPC recommends a dose of 1 g b.d. for a creatinine clearance of 50–31 mL/min.

Did you find this information in the SPC? If not, now is a good time to practise finding information about dosage changes in renal impairment in SPCs.

Suggested revision points

- Use of creatinine clearance and eGFR – where would you use each of these?
- Factors that influence creatinine clearance
- Use of SPCs to quickly locate dose adjustments for renal impairment.

Scenario 8.7 Antibiotic treatment regimens for endocarditis

Format: Written station

Supporting material available to student: *BNF*, SPCs for benzylpenicillin, flucloxacillin, gentamicin, vancomycin and rifampicin injections

Time allowed: 15 minutes

Suggested years of study: Undergraduate years 3 and 4 or pre-registration.

Knowledge and skills tested

- Data retrieval from different sections of the *BNF* and SPCs
- Numeracy without use of calculator.

Task

A 24-year-old male patient on your ward has been diagnosed with endocarditis. The junior doctor approaches you for advice about which antibiotics to prescribe. She describes the infection as 'severe' but explains that the causative bacteria are not yet known (although methicillin-resistant *Staphylococcus aureus* [MRSA] is not suspected). The patient does not have any allergies and has no previous history of cardiac problems. He weighs 66 kg. He has no renal or liver impairment

1. What advice would you give the doctor about which antibiotics to prescribe, the route of administration and appropriate doses in this patient?
2. What advice will you then give to the nurse on how to prepare and administer these antibiotics (note the ward does not stock ready-made doses)?

Scenario 8.7 feedback

1. What advice would you give the doctor about which antibiotics to prescribe, the route of administration and the appropriate doses in this patient?

Using the summary of antibacterial therapy table in the *BNF* (in section 5.1), the antibiotics of choice for initial 'blind' therapy are flucloxacillin and gentamicin. Referring to the individual monographs, the doses and routes are flucloxacillin 8 g in four divided doses (i.e. 2 g every 6 hours) by the IV route plus gentamicin 1 mg/kg (i.e. 66 mg) every 8 hours by IV route. Note that while the intramuscular (IM) route can be used, it would not be recommended in this case as the maximum flucloxacillin dose that can be administered in this way is 500 mg and multiple daily IM injections would be painful! Also, while some hospitals do not use 8-hourly gentamicin in endocarditis and have policies for this, an undergraduate would not be expected to know this!

2. What advice will you then give to the nurse on how to prepare and administer these antibiotics (note the ward does not stock ready-made doses)?

Using the *BNF*, flucloxacillin is available as 250 mg, 500 mg and 1 g vials. The student would be expected to recommend using 1 g vials. As per the flucloxacillin SPC, the nurse should reconstitute the 1 g vials with 15–20 mL water for injections then (back to *BNF*) add to 100 mL sodium chloride (NaCl) 0.9% or glucose 5% and give over 30–60 minutes.

Again using the *BNF*, gentamicin vials are 40 mg/mL (note the paediatric and intrathecal vials would NOT be appropriate). Thus the gentamicin concentration is 1 mg in 0.025 mL and 66 mg in 1.65 mL. Advise the nurse to draw up 1.65 mL of gentamicin 40 mg/mL (can use either 1 mL or 2 mL ampoules) and add to 50 or 100 mL NaCl 0.9% or glucose 5%. Administer over 20–30 minutes.

You would be expected to know that IV infusions should be used by the nurse rather than a slow IV injection. Slow IV injections are viewed as more of a risk to patients because of the potential for inadvertent rapid administration. Many hospitals only permit nurses to administer intravenous drugs by continuous or intermittent infusion.

Suggested revision points

- Routes of administration – definitions and uses of intramuscular injections, intravenous injections and intravenous infusions
- Empiric treatment of serious infections
- Clinical calculations without using a calculator
- Use of the *BNF* Appendix on intravenous additives.

Scenario 8.8 Ganciclovir infusion rate

Format: Written station

Supporting material available to student: *BNF*

Time allowed: 15 minutes

Suggested years of study: Pre-registration; postgraduate.

Knowledge and skills tested

- Data retrieval from *BNF*
- Practical aspects of administering infusions.

Task

A 38-year-old male patient on the admissions ward requires ganciclovir treatment for a newly diagnosed cytomegalovirus infection. He is immunocompromised as a result of medication he has been taking following his heart transplant last year. His current weight is 80 kg and his eGFR is 72 mL/min/1.73 m^2.

The on-call registrar asks you for advice on what dose to prescribe and to make a supply. Your pharmacy department stocks 250 mg in 100 mL pre-prepared infusion bags.

1. What dose, frequency, route and duration of therapy will you recommend?
2. What instructions will you give the ward staff on the volume of infusion that needs to be administered? If the infusion should be given over 1 hour, what rate (mL/min) should the pump be set at?
3. How many infusion bags will you supply to last from Saturday morning until Monday when the aseptics department can make an infusion containing the exact dose required?

Scenario 8.8 feedback

1. What dose, frequency, route and duration of therapy will you recommend?

As per *BNF*, initial treatment is 5 mg/kg (i.e. 400 mg) every 12 hours intravenously for 14–21 days. The student would not be expected to check the clinical appropriateness of ganciclovir other than it being used at an appropriate dose within its product licence.

2. What instructions will you give the ward staff on the volume of infusion that needs to be administered? If the infusion should be given over 1 hour, what rate (mL/min) should the pump be set at?

The ward will need 2 × 250 mg bags for each dose. A total dose of 400 mg needs 1 × 250 mg bag and 150 mg from the other bag.

So 250 mg in 100 mL means 1 mg in 0.4 mL and therefore 150 mg in 60 mL. Thus one full bag needs to be infused and 60 mL from the remaining bag.

If 400 mg in 160 mL is given over 1 hour then divide 160 by 60 to convert to mL/min.

The infusion should be run at 2.67 mL/min.

3. How many infusion bags will you supply to last from Saturday morning until Monday when the aseptics department can make an infusion containing the exact dose required?

Two bags are needed for each dose and five doses are needed in total (Saturday and Sunday morning and evening, Monday morning). Supply 10 bags.

You would be expected to know that special precautions need to be taken by personnel handling ganciclovir. Finally, on a practical note, you would be expected to make a supply to cover Monday morning so that the aseptics department are not under undue pressure to prepare the bag.

Suggested revision points

- Infusion devices and rates
- Cytotoxic infusions and handling out of hours requests.

Scenario 8.9 Co-trimoxazole dosage and administration

Format: Interactive station

Supporting material available to student: *BNF* and Septrin® for infusion SPC

Time allowed: 15 minutes

Suggested years of study: Pre-registration; postgraduate.

Knowledge and skills tested

- Data retrieval from different sections of the *BNF* and SPC
- Practical aspects of administration of infusions.

Task

You are the on-call pharmacist on a Sunday night. The intensive care unit (ICU) contact you about a female patient.

Mrs J, with *Pneumocystis jiroveci* pneumonia. She is 59 years old, weighs 96 kg, has renal impairment (eGFR 38 mL/min/ 1.73 m²) and is fluid restricted. The on-call registrar is just prescribing the co-trimoxazole infusion and wants to check the dose and how to administer it. The ICU has a stock of 10 × 5 mL ampoules of co-trimoxazole. Note that Mrs J has no known allergies.

1. What is an appropriate dose of co-trimoxazole and what frequency would you recommend? Justify your answer.
2. What volume of co-trimoxazole IV infusion is needed per dose, what diluent should it be added to and what is the total volume of each infusion that will be given to Mrs J?
3. How many 5 mL ampoules will you need to supply to ensure the ICU has enough to last 24 hours? Explain your answer.

Scenario 8.9 feedback

1. What is an appropriate dose of co-trimoxazole and what frequency would you recommend? Justify your answer

The SPC recommends 120 mg/kg in two or more divided doses (the *BNF* recommends 2–4 divided doses for 14–21 days). This means 120 × 96 = 11 520 mg daily for Mrs J.

In order to decide on dosage frequency you need to balance frequency of administration against nursing time and ease of preparation. You could recommend 5760 mg twice daily, 3840 mg three times daily or 2880 mg four times daily, but you would be expected to explain why (e.g. twice daily to minimise number of infusions needed). Looking at the volume of diluent needed, it is difficult to justify a three times daily dose as this is harder to reconstitute.

2. What volume of co-trimoxazole IV infusion is needed per dose, what diluent should it be added to and what is the total volume of each infusion that will be given to Mrs J?

The following diluents could be used: glucose 5%, or NaCl 0.9%. More options are listed in the SPC. The calculation below uses glucose 5% as an example, and is based on SPC advice for a fluid-restricted patient.

Each 1 mL injection contains 96 mg.

For a twice daily dose:

5760 ÷ 96 = 60 mL

Add each 5 mL co-trimoxazole to 75 mL glucose 5%

60 ÷ 5 = 12

12 × 75 mL = 900 mL

900 + 60 = 960 mL per infusion

For a three times daily dose:

3480 ÷ 96 = 40 mL

Add each 5 mL co-trimoxazole to 75 mL glucose 5%

40 ÷ 5 = 8

8 × 75 mL = 600 mL

600 + 40 = 640 mL per infusion

For a four times daily dose:

2880 ÷ 96 = 30 mL

Add each 5 mL co-trimoxazole to 75 mL glucose 5%

30 ÷ 5 = 6

6 × 75 mL = 450 mL

450 + 30 = 480 mL per infusion

3. How many 5 mL ampoules will you need to supply to ensure the ICU has enough to last 24 hours? Explain your answer

The answer is the same regardless of the frequency of administration, because full ampoules are used in this case.

Using the twice daily dose to illustrate:

11 520 ÷ 96 = 120 mL co-trimoxazole needed

120 ÷ 5 = 24 × 5 mL ampoules needed in 24 hours

Pack size of 10 × 5 mL ampoules and ICU have a stock of 10 already

You need to explain what you will supply. The easiest is 2 or 3 full packs (can expect ICU to use their existing stock or decide to ensure their stock is protected). Students can dispense part packs if they choose. Credit would be given for each response if it is explained.

Suggested revision points

■ Administration of medicines in fluid restricted patients
■ Sizes of commercially available infusion bags.

Scenario 8.10 Prednisolone reducing dosage

Format: Written station

Supporting material available to student: *BNF*

Time allowed: 10 minutes

Suggested years of study: undergraduate years 1–2.

Knowledge and skills tested

■ Numeracy without use of calculator.

Task

Mr D is being discharged home from hospital today after experiencing an exacerbation of his COPD (chronic obstructive pulmonary disease). He has completed a 10-day course of prednisolone 40 mg mane today and his discharge prescription instructs him to take 35 mg each morning for one week then reduce by 5 mg every week to zero.

1. How many 5 mg tablets will you need to supply to exactly cover his full reducing regimen?
2. Prednisolone 5 mg tablets are stocked as packs of 28 in your hospital. How many packs will you need?

Scenario 8.10 feedback

1. How many 5 mg tablets will you need to supply to exactly cover his full reducing regimen?

35 mg dose = 7 tablets $\times$ 7 days = 49

30 mg dose = 6 tablets $\times$ 7 days = 42

25 mg dose = 5 tablets $\times$ 7 days = 35

20 mg dose = 4 tablets $\times$ 7 days = 28

15 mg dose = 3 tablets $\times$ 7 days = 21

10 mg dose = 2 tablets $\times$ 7 days = 14

5 mg dose = 1 tablet $\times$ 7 days = 7

$49 + 42 + 35 + 28 + 21 + 14 + 7 = 196$ tablets

2. Prednisolone 5 mg tablets are stocked as packs of 28 in your hospital. How many packs will you need?

$196 \div 28 = 7$ full packs

Suggested revision points

- Examples of drugs used in high doses where patients routinely have to take multiple daily tablets.
- Reasons for reducing regimens of corticosteroids.

Scenario 8.11 Vitamin E dosage and administration

Format: Written station

Supporting material available to student: *BNF for Children*

Time allowed: 15 minutes

Suggested years of study: Undergraduate years 3, 4.

Knowledge and skills tested

■ Data retrieval from BNF for children
■ Interpretation of FP10 prescriptions.

Task

You receive an FP10 prescription in your pharmacy.

The details on the prescription are:

Title, Forename, Surname and Address: Miss Isabella Wright, 50 Mersey Avenue, Anytown A1 2BB
Age: 1 year
Number of days' supply: 28
Medication details: Vitamin E suspension 5 mL daily.

The prescription is signed, and the prescriber's details are present and correct. The prescription is in date.

You need to check the dose is appropriate and ask for Isabella's weight and the condition being treated. Isabella's mum tells you she has a rare condition called abetalipoproteinaemia which is looked after by the local Children's Hospital and that her weight is 23 pounds. Upon ringing the hospital, you find out that a dose of 50 mg/kg daily was intended.

1. What is Isabella's weight in kg?
2. Using this weight, what dose of vitamin E suspension is appropriate and are you happy to dispense the prescription? Explain why.
3. If you supply the vitamin E suspension at the dose prescribed by the GP, what volume is needed?

Scenario 8.11 feedback

1. What is Isabella's weight in kg?

You can use the weight conversion charts in the back of the *BNF* to answer this or work it out long-hand. There are 2.2 pounds in 1 kg, so $23 \div 2.2 = 10.45$ kg. Using the charts in the *BNF* will give you weight of 10.44 kg.

2. Using this weight, what dose of vitamin E suspension is appropriate and are you happy to dispense the prescription? Explain why

$$10.45 \times 50 = 522.7 \text{ mg daily dose}$$

The 5 mL dose prescribed is 500 mg daily which is straightforward to administer because the suspension is 500 mg in 5 mL. The 522.7 mg dose could be rounded to be given via an oral syringe to 525 mg (5.25 mL), which would not be as easy for mum to administer. Students would get marks for justifying whichever action they deemed best – either getting the prescription changed or allowing rounding down until Isabella's weight increased enough to round the dose up to the next sensible volume.

3. If you supply the vitamin E suspension at the dose prescribed by the GP, what volume is needed?

Note that the prescription asks for a 28-day supply to be made, so days required × volume:

$$28 \times 5 = 140 \text{ mL}$$

Suggested revision points

- Use of 'number of days supply' box on FP10s
- Use of oral syringes in babies and children.

Scenario 8.12 Dobutamine infusion rate

Format: Written station

Supporting material available to student: *BNF*

Time allowed: 10 minutes

Suggested years of study: Pre-registration; postgraduate.

Knowledge and skills tested

- Data retrieval from different sections of the *BNF*
- Practical aspects of syringe pump administration.

Task

One of the nurses on your ward asks you to help him with a calculation he needs to carry out before setting up a dobutamine infusion for one of your patients. Mr F, 73 kg, is on day 2 of a dobutamine infusion which is to be run at 4 micrograms/kg/minute through a central line. The nurse has got out a dobutamine 50 mL vial and the ward is using a 50 mL syringe pump.

1. What dose of dobutamine does Mr F need to receive every hour?
2. What infusion rate in ml/hour should the pump be set at?

Scenario 8.12 feedback

1. What dose of dobutamine does Mr F need to receive every hour?

4 micrograms/kg/minute needed

$4 \times 60 = 240$

So 240 micrograms/kg/hour needed

240 × 73 = 17 520 micrograms per hour or 17.52 mg.

2. What infusion rate in ml/hour should the pump be set at?

In the *BNF*, 50 mL vial contains 5 mg/mL and can be given undiluted:

17.52 ÷ 5 = 3.5 mL per hour (rounded down from 3.504).

Suggested revision points

■ Use of syringe pumps.

Chapter 8 feedback summary

In Chapter 8 you have looked at a whole range of practice situations involving calculations. These have included calculating the quantity to supply, conversions to different formulations

Table 8.1   Chapter 8 learning outcomes

Knowledge and skills	More work required	Feel competent
Extract key data in order to correctly solve a calculation problem		
Use formulae to manipulate data presented in a pharmacy situation		
Identify appropriate reference sources to use in different situations		
Retrieve information efficiently and explain this information effectively		

of the same products, drug dosages, administrations of intra-venous medication.

Now that you have completed this chapter, assess your competence in the knowledge and skills listed in Table 8.1. Jot down any notes that may help you.

If there are any points that you consider need further work, start a CPD (continuous professional development) cycle now to identify how you can achieve this action.

References and further reading

Rees JA, Smith I, Smith B (2005). *Introduction to Pharmaceutical Calculations*, 3rd edn. London: Pharmaceutical Press.

Summaries of Product Characteristics. Available from: www.medicines.org.uk/emc (accessed 11 June 2012).

Index

Note: Page references in bxx refer to boxes; fxx refer to Figures; and those in txx refer to Tables